ETHICAL ISSUES

Perspectives for the Physiotherapist

The only tyrant I accept in this world is the still voice within.

- M.K Gandhi

ETHICAL ISSUES

Perspectives for the Physiotherapist

Kavitha Raja
Fiddy Davis
Sivakumar T

PEEPEE
PUBLISHERS AND DISTRIBUTORS (P) LTD.

Ethical Issues

Published by
Pawaninder P. Vij

Peepee Publishers and Distributors (P) Ltd.
Head Office: 160, Shakti Vihar, Pitam Pura
Delhi-110 034 (India)

***Corporate Office:* 7/31, Ansari Road, Daryaganj**
Post Box-7243, New Delhi-110002 (India)

Ph: 55195868, 9811156083

e-mail: peepee160@yahoo.co.in

e-mail: peepee160@rediffmail.com

e-mail: peepee160@gmail.com

www.peepeepub.com

First Edition: **2006**

ISBN: 81-88867-80-2

Printed at:
Lordson, C-5/19, Rana Pratap Bagh, Delhi-110 007

Preface

The time is always right to do what is right
Dr. Martin Luther King Jr.

Ethics derives from the Greek word ethicos which means arising from custom; or from the French word ethos meaning custom. Websters's dictionary gives the meaning of the word as that which deals with moral issues of good and bad, based on societal norms. Staedman's medical dictionary defines medical ethics as the science of morality; the principles of proper professional conduct concerning the rights and duties of the health care professional, his patients and his colleagues.

With the above definition it is easy to see that it is rather difficult to draw up norms of behaviour as these will vary from situation to situation, country to country and often within the same country. This book aims to work only as a guide and by no means purports to be the gospel truth. The professional has to use his/her own judgment and reach his/her own conclusions. The authors do not attempt to give answers rather to pose questions in perspective. If after reading this book the professional is left with more questions than answers, our objective has been fulfilled.

However we feel that it is of great importance to have a book that outlines existing norms and gives at least some insight into the moral dilemmas that a practicing PT in this country is faced with. This book is meant for the student therapist or those therapists who are fresh graduates.

Although the main focus of the book is on clinical practice, we have touched upon academics and research as well as those issues that are facing the PTs of India today like the lack of a statutory regulatory body and the proliferation of distance education.

As this subject forms a part of the curriculum of the post graduate students and in some universities of the undergraduate students we felt it was necessary to have a book that encapsulates the subject. Hence this book. It is our hope that it meets at least some of the needs of the professional community.

Throughout this book the therapist will be referred to as "she" and the patient/ client as "he". This is merely to avoid confusion. We acknowledge the fact that there are a large number of men in this country who are practicing the science and art of physiotherapy with competence and dedication.

Terms such as health provider and client have been used as we acknowledge the fact that it is no longer a therapist- patient situation always. Normal individuals are increasingly seeking physiotherapeutic services for improved health and not just dysfunction.

The examples given are that of hypothetical situations only and any resemblance to actual episodes is purely coincidental. Furthermore, none of the clinical examples, is based on actual information on the subject.

Author

Contents

Chapter one

Introduction

Ethics is not definable, is not implementable, because it is not conscious; it involves not only our thinking, but also out feeling.

—Valdemar W. Setzer

What is Ethics?

Ethics derives from, the Greek word "ethicos" which means arising from custom or from the French word "ethos" meaning custom. According to Websters's dictionary ethics is a concept that deals with moral issues of good and bad, based on societal norms.

How should we live? Should we choose our happiness above all else? Is it right to live in luxury when others are suffering? If forced to follow laws that are against our principles, how should we react? These are questions of ethical consideration. These questions arise at all levels of life and in practically all situations. Although ethics is part of philosophy, it is an all-embracing practical aspect of day to day life and enters into all branches of life. Yet it is not a factual science. Rather it has to do with applying broad principles of right and wrong into actual situations.

Ethics, is the code written or unwritten that guides the behaviour of human beings, in the context of different cultures and situations. This moral code may vary from society to society. However there are certain aspects that hold good in every situation. The application of these principles would be dependent on the person and the situation. In short it is a judgment call.

Let us consider some examples of ethical and unethical behaviour. *A milkman who adds water to his milk is practicing unethical behaviour. He is cheating his customers who have a certain expectation of him which he is not living up to.*

On the contrary, *a shopkeeper who takes extra care to store provisions in order to protect them from insects and rodents, is practicing ethical behaviour as he is living up to the expectations of his customers.*

Most situations however are not so clear cut. There are situations where there are conflicting situations which may make the differentiation between right and wrong unclear.

Let us consider this hypothetical situation:

A family employs a woman, Amina, to care for their elderly grandmother Bhargavi. The entire care of Bhargavi is entrusted to Amina. Amina is given the same status in the family as other family members. Bhargavi depends on her entirely and speaks with her freely including aspects of family finances. Over a period of time, Amina has won the trust of all and has become an inalienable part of the family. One day Bhargavi tells Amina that after her death, all the jewellery belonging to her as well as her considerable savings which are kept in the house will be made over to Amina. This statement was made in the presence of family members all of whom agreed without reservations.

A couple of months later, Amina's married daughter comes into some financial difficulties and asks her mother for a large sum of money. Amina feels awkward to request her employers for a loan. Instead she considers taking the money out of the savings of Bhargavi which is anyway meant for her.

If Amina takes the money from the lady's savings, is it ethically wrong? Yes. This is so, because although the money may eventually be hers, the understanding was that it would be made over to Amina after the death of Bhargavi. What could she do instead?

Amina could tell Bhargavi in confidence about her financial needs and request help.

Amina could ask Bhargavi or the family for a loan.

When asked for a loan, the family immediately recall the previous conversation and get suspicious. One of them remark that the financial difficulty is a made up situation in order to get money from the grandmother after which Amina may disappear. Bhargavi on the other hand is entirely in favour of giving her the money from her own savings as she would, to any other member of her family. But the family prevent her.

Is this ethical? No. While Amina was treated as a member of the family when all was well, she is alienated once she requests help. There is a breach of trust on the part of the family. The family is also impinging on the rights of their grandmother by preventing her from doing what she wishes to.

The above example is one of ethical behaviour in a social situation. Historically this tenet has been well recognised from the early times. The Vedas, possibly the earliest philosophical writings, outline the way people must live. Hence these are probably the oldest ethical guidelines in the world. Likewise the code of Hammurabi, the writings of Confucius, The Koran and the Ten commandments from the Old Testament are examples of ethical guidelines from ancient times. Major thinkers of the world like Buddha, the Jain teachers, Taoists, Plato, Aristotle etc also outline norms of behaviour.

To translate this concept of ethical behaviour, into professional behaviour requires certain rules of conduct. These may be laid down by professional bodies or may just be rules that are widely understood but not laid down as rules per se.

Professional Ethics

Ethical considerations in professional situations may be even more complicated than in social situations. In addition to moral behaviour, the professional has to consider the ramifications or results that his actions may have on himself and other members of his profession.

Ethical dimensions in professions are needed to:

1. have clear boundaries
2. have commonly accepted norms of behaviour
3. enhance respect within and outside the profession

4. protect the rights of the consumer/ client
5. protect the rights and privileges of the professional

When the profession that is in question, is a service provider e.g. health, legal, it becomes even more important to have a set of rules by which the professional will abide. Here the importance is more on the protection of the rights of the consumer. The consumer is often in distress and at the mercy of the professional. Hence, a strict code of conduct is necessary. On the other side of the coin, once the distressing situation is under control, the client may have 20/20 hindsight and hold the provider responsible for lapses which may have been unavoidable or at worst, acceptable. Hence it is necessary to have strict guidelines so that the professional may have the support of the law if falsely accused of neglect or abuse.

Bioethics or Medical Ethics

Both in Eastern and Western medicine, the physician was required to adhere to certain codes of conduct before embarking on his profession. The Manusmriti, the works of Confucious and the Hippocrates oath all have examples of these.

The major thinkers of modern bioethics in the western system of medicine have been notably Thomas Percival, and lately Thomas Beauchamp and Childress who championed the " four principles" approach to bioethics.

Four Principles

To bound the rules of ethical behaviour, it is logical to adhere to the four principles as championed by Beauchamp. These principles are:

Autonomy: this is arguably the first of the four principles. In a broad sense it encompasses the other three. What is autonomy in this context? Autonomy of the client/ patient to opt for or out of any treatment options is available to him. If the health provider is able to respect the client's right to autonomy, much of the ethical burden will be taken care of.

Beneficence: this is the duty of the health provider to ensure that the client in her care is assured of all the benefits of her professional knowledge to help the person overcome their dysfunction.

Justice: is the duty of the health provider to ensure that justice is done to the individuals in her care. This involves equal and unbiased care, respect for autonomy, and the duty to provide the correct information to the best of her knowledge if called upon by a court of law.

Non-maleficence: this goes back to the oldest principle of medical behaviour—do no harm. This principle may sometimes come at odds with the first principle of autonomy. However it is the health provider's duty to ensure that no harm is done to the best of her knowledge.

Although there is a body of work on ethics based on the four principles, this philosophy is not without its detractors. Some of the objections to the four principles are that

1. They are not systematically related to one another
2. There is no priority ranking
3. Autonomy and beneficence conflict
4. They do not apply to research ethics

When autonomy and beneficence or non-maleficence are in direct conflict with each other, what is the professional to do? Justice is often hard to apply strictly as real life situations are often not clear cut. The thinkers, who object to the four principles approach, advocate the casuistry approach to medical ethics. Casuistry means decisions must be based on a case-by -case basis. As situations vary, there can be no set rules of action or behaviour. For example, while the principle of distributive justice, dictates that scarce resources must not be wasted, is it right to deny options to a patient? There can be no set answer to this as the situation will dictate the right course of action.

Ethical debate has historically been based on the principles of religion. Moral conduct has always been governed with respect to the divine word. However it is now important that ethical issues be based on secular principles.

Staedman's medical dictionary defines medical ethics as the science of morality; the principles of proper professional conduct concerning the rights and duties of the health care professional, his patients and his colleagues.

Ethics in the healthcare context is the set of values that guides the behaviour of the healthcare professional with regard to his/her interaction with individuals under his/her care. However there are various aspects of ethical behaviour in the healthcare context, which deal with not only interaction but also legal issues, dispersion of information, education, research etc.

We shall deal with these aspects in the context of the physiotherapy profession in the following chapters.

ETHICAL PRACTICE OF PHYSIOTHERAPY

Definition

Ethics in physiotherapy can be defined as the moral code of conduct that defines the relationship between the therapist and her patient or client, and the therapist and other healthcare professionals based on mutual respect and trust.

How does this affect the Physiotherapist (PT)? Physiotherapy evolved from the nursing profession during the First World War. Initially, the role of the physiotherapist was that of an ancillary professional to assist the physician. That scenario has undergone a sea change and in many parts of the world now, the physiotherapist is an independent professional. With this change in the job characteristics, comes a change in moral responsibility as well. When functioning as an ancillary, the PT was required to follow orders verbatim without using her own discretion. Under those circumstances, the ethical responsibilities were also that of the consulting physician. With increasing autonomy, the PT is now called upon to make decisions regarding commencement or cessation of treatment, changes in treatment etc, without the luxury of falling back on the physician for guidance. Under certain circumstances, the PT may be legally responsible for the well being of the patients under her care.

The PT whether in the employment of others or in self employment, is bound by a moral code in much the same way as that of any other health care provider. This is the concept of responsibility both overt and covert towards the patient.

Let us consider the following example:

A child with cerebral palsy is referred to you for treatment at your private clinic. According to the parents, the referring physician told them that "Physiotherapy would make their child alright" You have the following options:

1. *You go along with the parents' perception of what the physician said, as he is your major referral source, but add that it could take years.*
2. *You tell the parents "your doctor does not know what he is talking about. Your child will never be alright".*
3. *You tell the parents "it will cost Rs 200 per session, if you can afford it, I will see your child and see what I can do".*
4. *You tell the parents "I believe you may have misunderstood the doctor. Physiotherapy will not make your child alright. What he meant was that, you require to do physiotherapy and for many years to improve the abilities of your child. What I can do, is I will teach you what to do and see you at intervals to guide you, and you can follow through at home.*

Of the responses listed above, the first three are unethical. The first is reinforcing a wrong idea and hence giving the parents false hope. This is akin to a criminal offence. There is also a selfish motive in not wanting to upset your major referee.

The second while probably truthful, is undermining the standing of another professional. It is also callous. Hence this response is unethical as well.

The third option while not giving an opinion, is basing your cooperation on money. This is unethical in both ways. Money being the motivator is wrong and not giving your honest opinion based on facts is also wrong.

The fourth option, is the best, the most sensitive and professional. You could probably improve this response by speaking to the physician and informing him of what you have offered the parents.

In response to your reply (4), the parents storm out of your clinic after insulting you. They return to the doctor who sents them back to you, after thoroughly endorsing your opinion and stating that you are the best therapist in the area. The parents return to you and apologise for their earlier outburst.

1. *You tell them politely that they can go elsewhere as your reputation has been damaged with their public scene and you feel antagonistic towards them. You give them the name of another therapist.*
2. *You accept their apology gracefully, and accept and treat the patient to the best of your ability.*

As a healthcare professional the most ethical thing for you to do is the second option. However, if you feel that you will be unable to care for the child which includes extensive interaction with the parents, in an empathetic and professional manner due to their earlier outburst, the first option is probably better.

Patient

In any sort of relationship, all parties are bound to some extent by mutual responsibility. This is the case in a patient- health provider relationship as well. While the health provider is bound by rules of ethical conduct, so also is the client/ patient. Frivolous law suits is a case in point. While the health provider is bound to provide the best care that he/she is able to, accidents or unforeseen circumstances do happen. This may not be due to negligence and prosecuting the provider in this case may not be productive in the least. With increase in frivolous lawsuits, the knee jerk reaction of providers is to practice defensively. This can sometimes cause less than optimum results to the patient at greater cost in length of time and or actual treatment costs.

Let us take the following example:

You apply a hot pack to a patient following strict guidelines. You tell him he should not go to sleep and give him the call bell. The department is very busy and you check on him periodically. Without your knowledge, the patient removes some of the towelling in order to get more heat and in the process gives himself a blister.

On top of that, he claims that you did not warn him of possible consequences and he lodges a complaint with the medical superintendent.

This situation is an example of a **frivolous complaint**. There has been no lasting harm done, and the patient is at least as much at fault as the therapist. **A frivolous complaint is a complaint where the cause or incidence of dispute maybe so negligible as to be irrelevant.**

Such incidents, while rarely requiring more than a letter of explanation to the medical superintendent, may however prompt you in the future to apply more padding than necessary, thus decreasing the effect. This is an example of **defensive practice**. **Defensive practice is where the therapist takes undue caution in performing the skills of her profession such that there is almost no chance of an accident that maybe considered as negligence.** However, this can be considered irresponsible as the therapist is not practicing to the best of her ability.

The Therapist as a Service Provider

In the current context, the therapist as much as any other healthcare professional is a provider of services. This is not unlike say a bank officer who is a service provider. Only the kind of service differs in that healthcare providers are bound by moral laws probably much more than others with the exception of justice providers. The reason for this is the greater moral responsibility of health care providers as outlined earlier. When a customer goes to a bank, he is usually in a frame of mind to seek information, analyse the information given and make a logical decision based on his needs. This may not be the case of a patient who seeks treatment. Often the patients, who come to a physiotherapist on a first contact basis, do so for reasons of pain or severe discomfort. In such situations, he may not be in the adequate frame of mind to seek, analyse options and to make a clear decision. Added to this is the burden of medical jargon that the layperson may not be familiar with.

Conflicting information from the therapist and the physician or say the therapist and the media, or the therapist and a friend or relative may all add to the confusion and preclude the patient from making a decision or encourage him to forfeit that right. Finally it may boil down to "*do whatever you want but make sure I get better*". Once the initial discomfort is gone, however the patient may go back on his initial instructions and challenge the appropriateness of treatment. This can cause unpleasantness and the therapist may be outraged that her best intentions have backfired.

Responsibilities to the Customer (Patient/Client)

In this context the therapist has certain responsibilities to adhere to, in order to serve the best interests of the client. Most important after the four principles is confidentiality, economics, and dissipation of knowledge.

Confidentiality

This is included in the "justice" part of the four principles. Maintaining confidentiality of the patients under your care is of paramount importance. Often unthinkingly, professionals engage in discussions of patient characteristics in public places or without need. This amounts to dehumanisation of the individual. While it is impossible for healthcare providers not to discuss patients, it is important to consider the following facts:

1. Discuss only aspects of the patient that are important to the treatment of the individual e.g. therapists may discuss that a patient is overweight and hence requires a specially made walker due to safety concerns. This discussion is perfectly justified in this case. However if the same comment of the patient's size was made derogatorily in respect to say the application of electrical stimulation to the face where the size of the patient has no clinical implication, it amounts to a breach of trust.

2. Discuss aspects of care only in a confidential atmosphere and as much as possible without use of the patient's name or other identification. In addition ensure that the discussion does not involve anyone who cannot contribute to the enhanced care of your patient.
3. Ensure that patient records are not deposited in places of public access.
4. Do not discuss one patient's condition (1) with another patient (2) without the consent of the first party. It is often necessary for PTs to discuss positive aspects of another patient with a similar disability in order to motivate patients. Prior permission from patient (1) should be obtained or even better would be to engage the two patients and their families in a mutual discussion after consent is obtained from both.
5. Sometimes it may be necessary to withhold information from members of the patient's family if so requested. As a rule it is only necessary for the provider to give information to the patient, or if the patient is a minor or otherwise incapable of understanding the information, then the guardian specified in documents. If other relatives or friends seek information, general comments like "he is better", " he is improving" etc may be given. If pressed, the therapist can feign ignorance of aspects not directly under her purview or direct the person to the patient or guardian.

Economics

This aspect gains importance in resource poor societies like India, where often the costs of medical treatment are borne by the patient or family. In these situations, it becomes important that the therapist weigh her treatment options judiciously. Unnecessary economic burden on the patient when the treatment outcome is questionable should be avoided. An example of this would be:

A patient comes to you with multiple joint pains. In order to give pain relieving modalities to all painful joints would cost the patient Rs. 360.00 per session.

The pain relieving modality you would recommend is hot packs. You could decrease the patient's economic burden by advising them that the same temporary benefit could be achieved by hot fomentation at home and the patient should return to you once the acute pain has subsided for exercise prescription.

This information would need to be given in a tactful and sympathetic manner and preferably with the knowledge of the physician so that there is no conflict of advice.

Dissipation of Knowledge

This falls under the principle of "autonomy". The patient has a right to information pertaining to his condition. If the best information that the therapist can give is that she does not know, then this must be conveyed to the patient. The patient also has the right to make an informed choice of treatment options available to him as also the right to change providers if he so wishes. It is the duty of the therapist to provide information of aspects directly under her purview, in a comprehensive manner in a language that the patient can follow.

The Therapist in the Canvas of the Healthcare Profession

How does the PT fit into the medical professions canvas? The physiotherapist and indeed many of the rehabilitation professions are in a unique position in the healthcare spectrum. Physiotherapy is one of the professions, where the provider spends an inordinate amount of time with the patient thus gaining rapport and trust. This also has the flip side. Due to the relationship that a PT has with her patient, she is often asked for her opinion on a variety of healthcare factors many of which may not come directly under her purview. While the easiest way out of this dilemma is to bounce the question to another professional usually the physician, this may cause the patient to suspect that she is not being honest with him and or is hiding some unpleasant fact. Obviously there is no magic answer to these situations. Under the guidelines outlined above, the therapist must take the best stand she can.

Understanding of Ethics by Society

Societal interpretation of ethics is based on tradition and culture. What is appropriate behaviour in one culture may not be so in another. In some cultures it is not inappropriate for a lady patient to be asked to undress by a male professional. However, in some others this may be considered as highly inappropriate and the "perpetrator" liable to be prosecuted for misconduct. Hence it is important to work within the rules of the society one is dealing with and not only one's own perception of the situation.

Need for Guidelines

Why do we need ethical guidelines?

There are certain norms of human behaviour that overrides the barriers of religion, nationality, culture and gender. There are other norms that may be unique to certain populations and situations. Hence it is important that guidelines be drawn up so that there is consensus on codes of behaviour.

Summary

Ethical dimensions in professions are needed to:

1. have clear boundaries
2. have commonly accepted norms of behaviour.
3. enhance respect within and outside the profession
4. protect the rights of the consumer/client.
5. protect the rights and privileges of the professional

   The four Principles of bioethics are autonomy, beneficence, non-maleficence and distributive justice.

   In addition to these, the therapist has a responsibility to maintain confidentiality, respect the patient's right to information and maintain decorum while dealing with other professionals.

   Ethical practice guidelines are required in addition to protection of the patient to protect the professional against litigation.

Chapter two

Legal Issues

In civilized life, law floats in a sea of ethics
- Earl Warren

The possibility of litigation makes it necessary for a professional to be aware of ethical guidelines of practice and responsibilities to the client. The client is protected from malpractice or negligent practice on the part of the professional, by the **consumer protection act**. This act was passed in the year 1986.

Although there are no reported cases of litigation against physiotherapists for negligence or malpractice, the Indian Association of Physiotherapists, in its official publication in 2000, stated that the physiotherapist in India is liable under the consumer protection act as any other health provider.

In this context it is important that the practicing physiotherapist be aware of the provisions of the act, the application of the act and legal issues associated with it.

Why was the Statute Enacted?

The consumer protection act was enacted in order to provide

Protection to the consumers
Settlement of consumer disputes
Establishment of consumer forums

Application of the Act

The act applies to all goods as well as services rendered, unless expressly exempted by a notification from the central government.

What is Medical Service?

Services rendered by doctors and hospitals are held under the jurisdiction of the Act. However, any service rendered free of charge or under a contract of personal service (as in the case of home visits at the express request of the patient) does not come under the ambit of the Act.

Who is a Consumer of Services?

Any person who hires services against consideration (payment or charge of some kind) is a consumer. The medical practitioner or hospital undertaking and providing paramedical services of any category or kind would fall, within the definition of "service" and a person availing of such service would be a "consumer" within the meaning of the Act. Hence such a hospital or practitioner cannot claim immunity from the provisions of the Act.

However, a patient undergoing treatment in a Government Hospital or Charitable Institution is not a "consumer" under the Act as services in such institutions are rendered free of charge.

This interpretation was delivered by the Madras High Court on 17/2/1994. Thus it would entail that a patient or client seeking treatment under a physiotherapist, is a consumer and thus protected under the Act.

What is Deficiency?

Under the Act, deficiency in relation to any service means any fault, imperfection, short-coming, inadequacy in the quality, nature and manner of performance which is required to be maintained under the law. When there are two schools of thought or there is insufficient evidence to prove the superiority of one treatment over the other, neither would be upheld by the hallmark of legality.

Rights of Patients as Consumers

Patients as consumers have the right to:

be protected against marketing of hazardous goods and services.

be informed about the quality, quantity, potency, purity, standard and price of goods and services

be assured access to a variety of goods and services at competitive prices.

be heard and be assured that the consumers' interests will receive due consideration at appropriate forums

seek redressal against unfair and unscrupulous practices.

Duties of Professionals

Health professionals have the following duties towards the consumer or patient:

provide services with a degree of professional skill and expertise as would be expected from professionals of similar qualifications and standard.

provide services based on sound scientific principles

provide information on nature of disease, treatment and implications

not neglect a patient on personal grounds

informed consent for all invasive procedures.

Legal Duty

Whenever a person approaches another, trusting her to possess certain skill, or special knowledge on a given problem and depends on him for service and dispensation of that skill, she is bound under an implied legal duty. This legal duty dictates that she should exercise due diligence as is expected of her peers in the profession. This expectation is the least expected skill for the qualification that she possesses. Failure on the part of the professional to discharge service with the minimum competence expected, is tantamount to negligence and a breach of professional and legal duty.

Negligence

Negligence is an adverse event that occurs due directly to the lack of a reasonable degree of care or skill of the professional concerned. Mere error of judgement does not amount to negligence unless the error is of such a kind that no average or ordinary physiotherapist would commit it. For example, if no ordinary physiotherapist would give treatment of diathermy to a pregnant lady, it would be negligence if some physiotherapist gives such a treatment. But if there is a difference of opinion prevailing among the profession, and a considerable number of therapists are of the view that such treatment can be given, then it would not be considered as negligent behavior or malpractice.

Vicarious Liability

Vicarious liability is the legal responsibility placed on a person when that person takes the place of another as far as liability is concerned. For example, the liability of a hospital extends to the actions of its employees. Similarly, the liability incurred by a junior member of the staff or an aide or attendent, extends to the senior member of staff.

If a physiotherapy aide whose job description includes assisting therapists with application of wax bath, inadvertently causes a burn, the liability ensued is that of the supervising therapist and not of the aide.

This is because, although the actual act was performed by the aide, his training and knowledge precludes him from responsibility for the effects that may ensue. Moreover, the supervising therapist has the responsibility to assess and ensure that the treatment given is appropriate and safe.

Redressal Mechanism under the Act

Disputes that arise that fall under the Act will be adjudicated at the district, state and national levels. The **district consumer disputes redressal forum** is established in each district by the state government. Then there is the **state consumer disputes redressal commission** established by the state government. Finally there is the **national consumer disputes redressal commission** established by the central government.

The burden to prove that the physiotherapist was negligent is upon the complainant. However, if the facts are so obvious that negligence can be easily inferred to, then the burden shifts upon the physiotherapist to prove that she was not negligent and that she had exercised reasonable care and skill. For example, if a patient were to have burns as a result of application of hot packs, it would be up to the physiotherapist to show that there was no negligence and such burns are one of the risks of the treatment as was explained to the patient.

Although most of the litigations deals with medical practitioners it can be safely said that the same standards would be applied by the courts in case of physiotherapists.

Compensation

Damages, compensation and other incidental reliefs are based on certain well established principles. There are certain tables and schedules according to which the quantum of compensation is awarded. This includes life expectancy, capacity to earn, potential loss in case of physical disability, grief etc. Although each case is unique, the quantum of compensations is made commensurate with the degree of dereliction. Incidental costs are also covered. There is no guarantee that whatever is claimed will be awarded.

The following factors are considered as supporting and sometimes mitigating circumstances

a. Nature and degree of loss- gravity of the injury and the period that it would persist
b. Implications that would arise form the injury in day to day life
   i. Financial implications
   ii. Mental agony
   iii. Social embarrassment
   iv. Survival of dependents
c. Age of the patient
d. Source of income
e. Prospects for career
f. Detriment caused due to the disability
g. Other co morbid conditions
h. Concept of contributory negligence.

Safeguards

Preventive and remedial measures available to physiotherapists to avoid or minimise the risk of litigation:

a. If the services are rendered without charging any money, "Free consultation" must be mentioned on the prescription and the signature of the patient obtained; as free services are exempt from the provisions of the Act.
b. The patient must be informed about the necessity of treatment, its alternative modalities and duration, the inherent risks to which the patient may be exposed to, whether such risks are a direct result of treatment and the expenses and its break up. In other words an informed consent must be obtained.
c. The methods used must always be those that are recognised and approved by practitioners who are reasonably skilled in the profession.
d. The therapist must always obtain professional indemnity insurance
e. Before taking any decision as to the line of treatment to be given, the therapist must adopt all precautionary procedures. For example, it is always necessary to follow universal precautions.

Some examples of litigation are given below:

Q1. *I have instituted a complaint before the Consumer Court against a Medical Practitioner. My complaint has been challenged on the ground that a Medical Practitioner cannot be sued under the Consumer Act. What does law provide?*

Ans. *Yes, a medical practitioner can be sued under the Consumer Protection Act 1986 for his or her professional negligence resulting in damage to patient. Section 2 (d) in defining a consumer in Clause (ii) uses the expression 'hires and avails of". The word "hire" means employ of wages or fees". Secondly the words "any service" in s. 2 (d) (ii) in Consumer Protection Act. brings the delinquent medical practitioners within the ambit of Consumer Protection Act. Thirdly, s. 2 (o),*

Consumer Protection Act which defines service exempts only two types of services, one "service free of charge" and another "contract of personal service" which postulates a relationship of master and servant. A medical man whose service is requisitioned for a patient answers the clause " contract of service" but never "a contract of personal service". So, a negligent medical professional can be litigated under the Consumer Protection Act 1986.

Q.2. *I injured my knee in a game of football on 31st December 1997. It was diagnosed as ACL TEAR. For that I was operated upon in the knee on 2nd March 1998. After the operation my knee developed stiffness, which is unusual in such cases. Even after undergoing physiotherapy for two months I was unable to bend or straighten my knee. So after two months of operation my knee was manipulated under anesthesia to relieve stiffness. A plaster was put on the knee for one month. I was told to start walking . I used to walk with a limp. For about 8 months I continued to walk with a limp but then my condition deteriorated & in March-99 I had to start using crutches to move around. To find out the cause of this pain I underwent investigative arthoscopy in June-99 which revealed the following 1. ACL Laxity 2. meniscus tear 3. patellofemoral osteo-arthritis. I was advised by the doctor to do physiotherapy, and take painkillers for the pain, I am still doing physiotherapy, but neither has the pain reduced nor am I able to walk without crutches. This whole experience has affected my life badly. Can I sue the doctors for negligence / inefficiency. Both operations were carried out in military hospitals, and they were done free of cost since I am serving in army. So can I go to Consumer protection court. Please advise?.*

Ans. *You can file a written petition in the High Court against the hospital, making doctors responsible for your condition liable. You can also seek* *damages along with the appropriate action against the doctors and the management in the written petition*

In the second example, it is highly possible for the physiotherapist to be held liable as well. However, since the situation is one of a hospital, it is more likely that the hospital and the surgeon will be held liable vicariously. Now again, it is highly likely that the patient had not followed instructions after his several operations and thus developed stiffness. So the burden to prove that the professionals were at fault rests with him.

One of the important landmarks in disability legislation in India is The Persons With Disability (PWD) Act of 1995. The importance of this act is that it is the first comprehensive legislation which addresses the rights of the disabled population. This act is also called the Equal Opportunities, Protection of Rights and Full Participation Act. The act was passed in order to empower the disabled among our population. It lays down norms for barrier free architecture as well as concessions and provisions for the disabled.

With the popularity that "health tourism" is enjoying, there are certain aspects of international agreements that the physiotherapist must be aware of. These may have an indirect application in the physiotherapist's practice. The reasons are more cultural but they may eventually have legal implications especially in the areas of informed consent.

The GENERAL AGREEMENT ON TRADE IN SERVICES (GATS) is the first set of international rules for the international trade in services. India has been a signatory to the Agreement since 1995. GATS sets out a framework of legally-binding rules governing the conduct of world trade in services. The GATS applies in principle to all service sectors except "services supplied in the exercise of governmental authority",

The GATS sets out four modes of supplying services. Of these the first three are relevant to the physiotherapist.

Mode 1 Cross-border trade corresponds with the normal form of trade in goods and maintains a clear geographical separation between seller and buyer. In this case services flow from the territory of one member into the territory of another member crossing national frontiers. Telemedicine is an example of this.

Mode 2 Consumption abroad refers to situations where a service consumer moves into another member's territory to obtain a service (e.g. consumer travelling for tourism, medical treatment, to attend educational establishment).

Mode 3 Commercial presence is the supply of a service through the commercial presence of the foreign supplier in the territory of another WTO member. In this case a service supplier of one member establishes a territorial presence in another member's territory to provide a service. (E.g. the establishment of branch offices or agencies to deliver such services as banking, legal advice or communications or education).

Health Services and Social Services

Medical and Dental services, services provided by midwives, nurses, physiotherapist, paramedical personnel, hospital services and other human health services social services are covered under this. India has been requested to allow the following for doctors, dentists, midwives, nurses, physiotherapists and paramedical personnel:

take full market access and national treatment commitments in Modes 1,2 & 3 .

allow joint ventures

permit foreign doctors with national licences in the country of origin to practice for three years or more.

In turn India has made similar requests to other member countries.

take full market access and national treatment commitments in Modes 2 & 4 for medical and dental services, services provided by midwives, nurses, physiotherapists, and paramedics.

create a visa system to ensure the access as per commitments made.

It is conceivable that, in the future, physiotherapists may be accountable for their actions under the legal system. The borders that bound what is "reasonable" may undergo a change with increase in awareness and cross cultural influences. Hence it is important that legal and ethical guidelines be adhered to in practice at all times.

Summary

The Consumer Protection Act of 1986 is applicable in cases of complaints against medical practitioners. It outlines the responsibilities of the service provider. The following steps can be taken by the professional as safeguards against litigation:

- Indemnity insurance
- Informed consent
- Guidelines of practice.

Chapter three

International Organizations and their Regulations

Ethics must begin at the top of an organisation. It is a leadership issue and the chief executive must set the example.

—Hennessey

Physiotherapy is being practiced widely in all countries as an adjunct to medical care for patients with selected dysfunctions. To guide the physiotherapist in moral and ethical issues each country has levied some legal responsibilities through governing bodies which the physiotherapist is expected to adhere to without any compromise. The governing body of each country is a member of the World Confederation for Physical Therapy (WCPT). The World Confederation for Physical Therapy, which was founded in 1951 to represent physical therapists internationally, champions the principle that every individual is entitled to the highest possible standard of culturally-appropriate health care provided in an atmosphere of trust, respect for human dignity, underpinned by sound clinical reasoning and scientific evidence. The Confederation is a non-profit organization comprising 92 member organizations which, together, represent more than 250,000 physical therapists worldwide. WCPT undertakes a range of programs and projects and supports international campaigns, which promote the physical therapy profession and its contribution to global health. It encourages high standards of physical therapy research, education and practice and maintains official relationships and strategic alliances with government and non-government agencies worldwide, including the World Health Organization. WCPT provides governments, regulatory bodies and other professional groups with background information about the professional nature of physical therapy (More details in Appendix).

The ethical principles are formed according to the culture and attitude of the clients and the physiotherapists. The governing body has a responsibility to the members of the society served by the profession and also to the profession. It attempts to fulfill its responsibility by requiring its members to adhere to certain ethical principles and standards of conduct.

Need to Know International Regulations

Give us an insight about the moral practice principles in other countries

Guide physiotherapists who are aspiring to work overseas about the legal and moral responsibilities they need to know

Give an idea about how to change our ethical principles with content validity and make our profession transparent as other professions.

Even though all the ethical principles and legal responsibilities can be categorized in our four principles of Autonomy, Beneficence, Justice and Non – maleficence, we need to consider specific instances. What is considered ethically unacceptable in one country may be acceptable in another e.g. Poor/inadequate documentation.

The governing bodies in all countries have a panel of members who will assess not only the morality of physical therapy care administered to the clients but also the responsibilities of the physical therapist to the profession and her personal development. The American Physical Therapy Association (APTA) has an Ethics and Judicial Committee (EJC) which watches its members for ethical behavior.

There are a variety of issues addressed by the governing bodies about ethical behavior and morality. In this chapter we will be dealing with issues which need special emphasis and issues which are not commonly dealt with in India.

Advertising

It is ethical for a physiotherapist to advertise physical therapy products and services provided that they:

Exercise sound professional judgment.

Disclose any financial interest in the distribution of product and services.

Abide by any legal restrictions affecting such endorsements.

Avoid the appearance of endorsement from the governing bodies. (APTA)

Advertisement whether written or audio-visual, should not be false, fraudulent, misleading, deceptive, self-laudatory, unfair or sensational. This also applies to the use of qualifications and titles. It is undesirable (but not unethical) to use too many qualifications. Claims of superiority over other Practitioners in respect of personal skills, facilities or equipments must not be made

(Chartered Society of Physiotherapists)

APTA regularly adopts and publishes policies and positional statements. Some of these policies and statements contain ethical mandates.

Compensation for Referral and Patient Exploitation

APTA has published a statement on public policy position and a statement on ethical mandate for its members. It has taken a position opposing arrangements between referring practitioners and physical therapists where the referring practitioners benefit economically from the provision of services.

It is believed that introduction of financial incentives into the referral process unnecessarily increases the potential for abuse of that process. When the referring practitioners knows that he will derive income from the referred services, the possibility of over utilisation, for unnecessarily inflated costs and undue restriction for patients' autonomy will result.

Whenever the association contemplates action on this issue against a member which might affect her ability to practice, the association takes into account the antitrust ramifications of its action.

Documentation

Paper work is one of the least attractive professional responsibilities, especially in a busy clinical setting. Documentation is part of providing service and it is an ethical matter. Lack of proper documentation or inadequate record keeping is considered more than poor clinical practice.

Upon accepting an individual for the provision of physical therapy services, physical therapists are to assume responsibility for maintaining adequate records of the case including progress reports. APTA takes disciplinary action on its members who are involved in inadequate documentation or total lack of case records.

Sale of Services and Goods

Physiotherapist shall not sell, supply, endorse or promote the sale of services and goods in ways which exploit the professional relationship with patients.

Physiotherapists may sell, supply services and goods in clinical practice after they have satisfied themselves that the item is appropriate for that particular patient. Physiotherapist should not accept commission from the third parties for recommending the purchase of goods and services (CSP).

Except for the remuneration to which he is entitled, a physiotherapist shall not receive, pay or undertake to pay any benefit, rebate or commission in connection with the practice of his profession (South African Society of Physiotherapy).

Inappropriate Relationship with Patients

The therapeutic relationship between the physiotherapist and patient must be based on mutual trust and respect. A Physiotherapist who exploits this relationship either within or outside the treatment environment is acting in contravention to this rule. Patients may also seek to exploit the relationship. The physiotherapist must be alert to any signs of this happening and take steps to restore appropriate interaction or to withdraw from the situation. It is forbidden for a physiotherapist to have sexual relations with the patient (CSP).

New Zealand society of Physiotherapists (NZSP) has categorized sexual harassment of varying degrees as:

Sexual Impropriety: any behavior or expressions such as gestures or expressions that is sexually demeaning to a patient or which demonstrate a lack of respect for patient's privacy

Sexual Transgression: includes any inappropriate touching of a patient that is sexual of nature and short of sexual violation

Sexual Violation: Physiotherapist/Patient sexual activity whether or not initiated by the Physiotherapist

Informed Choice and Consent

The physiotherapist ensures that patients are able to make an informed choice and give informed consent to the proposed physiotherapy interventions.

The physiotherapist must provide patients with sufficient information including significant benefits, risks and side effects of proposed treatments, in a manner they can understand in order to make an informed decision.

Patients have the right:

To discuss treatment during its course.

To voice any concerns about the state and quality of the service.

To withdraw from or refuse treatment at any stage. This must be accurately documented.

To ask about treatment alternatives and to be told what is available in a manner which they can understand (NZSP)

Informed consent demands that the patient understands in lay person terms, all the advantages and disadvantages of the proposed treatment regime. It may be practical to present a written explanation before the first contact as to what a patient may expect during assessment and treatment.

If patients are not provided as much information, as they reasonably need to make their decision, and in a form they understand, their consent may not be valid. At all stages of assessment and treatment it is essential that the physiotherapist is satisfied that valid consent has been obtained. Some procedures like self positioning need not have a written consent but consent by word of mouth can be obtained. The physiotherapist should document, when the consent is received, whether implied or expressed.

Even therapeutic touching that is without the consent of the patient comes within the scope of criminal offence of "Assault and Battery" and possible civil action of "Trespass to the person" Emergency treatment may exclude the possibility of a formal consent for example an acute painful condition or a sports field injury. (CSP)

Confidentiality

The physiotherapist treats all information provided by the patient as confidential and only divulges information with the patient's permission, except when the law requires otherwise.

The physiotherapist provides an appropriate level of personal privacy for patients.

Patient records must be securely stored at all times to prevent unauthorized access to patient information. (NZSP)

Information relating to the physical therapist / patient relationship is confidential and may not be communicated to a third party not involved in that patient's care without the prior consent of the patient (APTA)

In some cases patients are unaware of the diagnosis e.g. Carcinoma or a chronic degenerating neurological disorder such as Parkinson's disease or Multiple Sclerosis. Patients may be unsure as to why they have been referred to physiotherapy and ask the physiotherapist for a diagnosis. Such information must be given only by the health professional (in most cases it will be the patient's physician) who has overall responsibility for the patient. Rapid contact with the doctor to inform him / her that the patient is requesting this information is essential, if necessary indicating the dilemma faced by the physiotherapist with the patient who does not know the reason for referral to physiotherapy (CSP).

Professional Responsibility

A physical therapist shall make professional judgments that are in the client's best interests.

Regardless of practice setting, a physical therapist has primary responsibility for the physical therapy care of a patient and shall make independent judgments regarding that care consistent with accepted professional standards (APTA).

A physical therapist shall not provide physical therapy services to a client while her ability to do so safely is impaired (APTA).

A physical therapist shall exercise sound professional judgment based upon her knowledge, skill, education, training, and experience (APTA).

Upon accepting a client for physical therapy services, a physical therapist shall be responsible for: the examination, evaluation, and diagnosis of that individual; the prognosis and intervention; re-examination and modification of the plan of care; and the maintenance of adequate records, including progress reports. A physical therapist shall establish the plan of care and shall provide and/or supervise and direct the appropriate interventions (APTA).

If the diagnostic process reveals findings that are outside the scope of the physical therapist's knowledge, experience, or expertise, the physical therapist shall so inform the client and refer him to an appropriate practitioner (APTA).

When the patient has been referred from another practitioner, the physical therapist shall communicate pertinent findings and/or information to the referring practitioner (APTA).

A physical therapist shall determine when a client will no longer benefit from physical therapy services (APTA).

The physiotherapist identifies, discusses and formulates functional measurable treatment goals and outcomes in conjunction with the active participation of the patient (NZSP).

The physiotherapist only practices in those areas in which she is competent (NZSP).

Where a patient's needs lie outside the scope of the physiotherapist's expertise, the patient shall be informed and assisted in identifying a qualified person to provide the necessary services (NZSP).

The physiotherapist ensures that clinical practice does not conflict with any other known treatment the patient is receiving (NZSP).

The physiotherapist undertakes progressive reviews of clinical practice outcomes with the patient (NZSP).

The physiotherapist keeps the patient's referring health professional e.g. General practitioner informed of the patient's progress and any concerns the physiotherapist may have (NZSP).

The physiotherapist ceases intervention if the physiotherapy clinical practice does not achieve identified goals within a time frame appropriate to the condition or injury, or does not enable the patient to maintain health or lifestyle (NZSP).

The physiotherapist ceases intervention when the physiotherapy clinical practice has achieved and sustained agreed defined functional goals (NZSP).

A physiotherapist shall not sell or otherwise provide, for profit, articles or equipment necessary for rehabilitation and, in particular, crutches, canes, walkers or pharmaceutical products.

Contribution to the Advancement of the Profession

The physiotherapist must, as far as he is able, contribute to the development of his profession through the exchange of his knowledge and experience with his colleagues and students, and his participation in courses, scientific conventions and training periods.

Responsibilities to Society

1. Physiotherapists shall recognize their responsibility to improve standards of health care.
2. Physiotherapists shall comply with all laws and regulations pertaining to the practice of physiotherapy.
3. Physiotherapists shall report, to the appropriate authorities, any member of the profession who appears to be incompetent or whose conduct while practicing as a physiotherapist appears to be unethical or illegal.
4. Where a direct fee is charged, physiotherapists shall inform clients, in advance, of the fee which will be commensurate with the service provided.

(Canadian Physiotherapy Association)

Continuing Education and Personal Development:

The physiotherapist has a duty to keep up to date with professional skills and knowledge.

The physiotherapist maintains at all times the highest standard of professional practice and continues to update and extend her professional knowledge and skills. (NZSP)

The physiotherapist is aware of research and evidence based practice relevant to physiotherapy and improving patient management, and recognizes the need for ongoing research. (NZSP)

The physiotherapist keeps up to date with legislation relevant to the practice of physiotherapy. (NZSP)

The physiotherapist keeps up to date with appropriate management training. (NZSP)

The physiotherapist reads current literature on professional and clinical matters. (NZSP)

The physiotherapist is committed to personal development and continuing education by attending relevant courses, workshops, lectures and seminars (NZSP).

The physiotherapist recognizes the benefits of communication and exchange of ideas and information by networking within the physiotherapy profession and the wider health sector. (NZSP)

The physiotherapist participates in a peer review system appropriate to the workplace. (NZSP)

The Indian Association of Physiotherapists (IAP) is one of the member organizations in the World Confederation for Physical Therapy (WCPT). With the background information provided by the WCPT, IAP has formulated ethical principles and all physical therapists are expected to adhere to the same. Two of the important principles reinforcing this are:

Principle 2: Physical therapists must comply with the laws and regulations concerning the practice of physical therapy in the country in which they work.

Principle 5: Physical therapists are committed to providing quality services according to quality policies and objectives defined by their national physical therapy association.

Disciplinary Action

Any complaint with regard to professional misconduct can be brought before the regulatory body for disciplinary action. Upon receipt of any complaint of professional misconduct, the regulatory body would hold an enquiry and give opportunity to the physical therapist to be heard in person or by a pleader. If she is found to be guilty of committing professional misconduct the regulatory body may award such punishment as deemed necessary (withholding the license to practice) for a specific period or permanently. In India, IAP is neither authorized to conduct an enquiry nor stop physiotherapists (who are found to be guilty of committing professional misconduct) from practicing. In India all the hearings of professional misconduct will be done by the consumer forum. It is normally the practice to resort to the MCI guidelines in case of litigation against any health care professional. The role of MCI over these issues is not clearly defined, this could partly be because there are very few cases of professional misconduct among physiotherapists that come up for disciplinary action.

Summary

WCPT has broad guidelines for the practice of All member nations formulate laws based on these guidelines as well as the unique needs of the country. Knowledge of how other nations define ethics is necessary with globalisation.

Chapter four

Clinical Practice

If a man is good in his heart, then he is an ethical member of any group in society. If he is bad in his heart, he is an unethical member. To me, the ethics of medical practice is as simple as that.

- Dr Elmer Hess

First of all we shall take a look at what the "four principles" of bioethics means. This concept has been introduced in the first chapter.

As stated earlier the "four principles" are:

Beneficence

Autonomy

Distributive justice

Non-maleficence

To further explain these concepts:

Beneficence

This principle defines the duty of the health provider to practice in a way that benefits the patient or client under her care.

How do we ensure this?

In order to ensure that the patient has the greatest benefit from the treatment being provided to him, the therapist must be sure that

1. The treatment offered is the best available option
2. The treatment has the potential to improve the patient's condition
3. She has the knowledge, facilities and skill to deliver the treatment in the optimum fashion

Autonomy

This principle defines the right of the patient to choose the treatment offered to him and includes his right to refuse any treatment option he may consider as useless or harmful or otherwise. The patient also has the right to choose his therapist or refuse a particular therapist.

Hence in order to respect the autonomy of the patient the therapist must be able to

1. Outline treatment choices and any benefits or harmful effects if the patient seeks this information
2. Gracefully hand over care to another therapist if the patient so wishes
3. Not use coercion or other forms of force to make a patient comply with treatment

Distributive Justice

This principle came into the forefront when haemodialysis machines were first introduced. As the machines were few, the physicians had no choice but to pick those patients who had the greatest chance of survival. Fortunately, such life saving decisions rarely confront physiotherapists.

This principle defines the distribution of resources in a fair and just manner. In this context, it is generally agreed that "**the preferential option for the poor**" is justified. What this means is that when resources are few and have to be shared by many, the economically backward, the desperate, and the underprivileged be given preference. In addition, those that have greater number of dependents, small children may be given preference. However these situations generally arise in life saving options. Where the physiotherapist is concerned, such situations are unlikely to occur. Nevertheless, let us consider the following example:

A community physiotherapist has two economically backward paraplegics for whom she is trying to gain employment. A philanthropist comes forward and offers to employ one. The therapist is asked to recommend the one that she considers most suitable. Both of the patients are similar in age and education. However one is married with two small children and was the only earning member of the family before the accident. The other is unmarried and his father and brother are working and supportive.

By the principle of distributive justice, the obvious choice for the job would be the patient with the dependent children.

Non-maleficence

This principle defines the duty of the therapist to do no harm. In order to adhere to this principle, the therapist must:

1. Keep up-to-date with recent advances in the area.
2. Gain adequate information from the patient prior to treatment
3. Seek any information that may be missing from the file and is of relevance
4. Opt for a harmless treatment when there is a doubt.

To elucidate with an example:

A young lady comes to the therapist for treatment of her low back pain. After the therapist assesses her, she decides to give her short wave diathermy. This is also in keeping with the physician's recommendation. The therapist gives her several sessions of treatment. During the course of conversation one day, the therapist discovers that the patient is 10 weeks pregnant. The therapist realizes that she had failed to ask her about the possibility of being pregnant before starting treatment.

This is a case where the principle of non-maleficence was not adhered to. This amounts to negligence as one of the standard questions to be asked prior to applying SWD is the possibility of pregnancy.

Another important aspect of non-maleficence, is the duty of the therapist to take precautions against illness or injury to the patients under her care. The rules of infection control is a case in point. Not adhering to the practice of "universal precautions" or using safety measures like wearing non slip shoes on the part of the therapist, puts the patients under her care at risk and thus constitutes inappropriate, irresponsible and hence negligent behaviour.

After the "four principles" come the next most important aspects of ethics during practice.

Confidentiality

Definition: confidentiality, is the act of maintaining secrecy pertaining to information concerning another individual. This can arguably fall under the principle of non-maleficence.

What does it mean in the patient-therapist relationship?

There maybe many aspects of the patients/ clients under her care that a physiotherapist must maintain confidentiality in. These aspects would be

1. Nature of medical affectation—this maybe especially important in cases where the medical affectation may have a negative impact as in questionable morals in the eyes of society e.g. AIDS, alcoholic neuropathy etc.
2. Prognosis—if the prognosis is questionable, there maybe ramifications that would affect the family and the individual's care e.g. withdrawal of necessary care due to economic burden for a high level paraplegic by the family.
3. Nature of treatment—this maybe more so in invasive procedures rather than with physiotherapy. The exact nature of treatment may cause conflict with certain beliefs which may aid to social isolation. e.g. blood transfusion in case of Jehovah's witnesses.
4. Cost of treatment—unless the person seeking information is directly responsible for payment of costs towards treatment, this information need not be divulged to anyone seeking information.

Many patients and their families do not appreciate outsiders prying into the specifics of their condition. At the least, it can be a nuisance and an invasion of privacy. Hence it is important that therapists take care when discussing aspects of patient care in open or public places. It is always better to discuss specifics in a closed room with only the relevant individuals present. Often due to the construction of physiotherapy departments it is difficult if not impossible to maintain strict confidentiality. Also, as mentioned earlier, it is frequently in the best interests of concerned patients to have group interaction between patients with the same diagnosis. This often acts as a stimulus for increased patient participation. So how do we maintain confidentiality? It would be necessary for the therapist to first get the consent of the individuals involved before she gets them into groups. The other strategy that she can employ when questioned about another patient's condition is to bounce the question back saying "I am not allowed to discuss details of patients with others. However I have no objection to you asking him personally". When requesting permission from patients to discuss aspects of their care with other patients, specifics of the permission must be obtained. e.g. is it permissible to discuss mode of injury and prognosis? Or are there aspects that they would rather the therapist do not discuss.

Another aspect of confidentiality, involves health providers discussing patients among themselves. This forms the greater and more widespread issue than therapist-patient discussions. It is almost impossible for therapists to refrain from discussing patients and their conditions and characteristics. As therapists spend a great deal of time with their patients, it becomes difficult not to form opinions about them. Care must be taken to ensure that names and other identifying factors are not talked about in the hearing of others.

The other greatest threat to confidentiality is the misplacement of written patient notes. Patient notes form part of the medical file which is a legal document. Care must be taken that all patient notes are in the appropriate sections in the medical file and fastened according to the procedure practiced.

Why is it necessary?

Confidentiality is necessary for the following reasons:

1. To protect the patient/ client from an invasion of their privacy
2. To protect the professional from unwarranted litigation
3. To respect the individuality of the patients under the therapist's care.

What does a breach of confidentiality mean?

A breach of confidentiality is when the therapist knowingly or inadvertently, discloses information of a confidential nature to another individual or individuals without authorization from the patient or client. This does not hold good if the therapist is required to disclose any information sought by a court of law. Also if the information may have life saving potential it is permissible. Let us consider the following example:

A patient who is very depressed due to chronic pain in the joints, talks about suicide once or twice. He tells the therapist not to mention it to his family as they would be upset.

It would be in the best interest of both the family and the patient, if the therapist mentioned this conversation with his family. It may help them seek psychiatric care for the patient's depression, or in other ways be more empathetic and improve the quality of the patient's life. A breach of confidentiality here is justified.

A patient the therapist is treating is HIV positive. He requests the therapist to conceal this information from his wife.

It would be against the principle of non-maleficence if the therapist did not disclose this information to his wife. Hence a breach of confidentiality is justified.

Right to make informed choices

This falls under the principle of "autonomy".

Definition: autonomy is the right of an individual to decide for himself/ herself the course of action to be followed.

Obviously for a patient to exercise this right, they must have sufficient knowledge of what is involved. This is where the issue of "informed consent" applies. This is discussed in detail in the second chapter.

What does it mean in the patient-therapist relationship?

Respect for the patient's right to autonomy: respect for autonomy is the moral obligation to respect the right of others to have opinions that may be contrary to your own. This should be compatible with the respect for all those potentially affected in the same manner. What this means is that the therapist should have a set of moral guidelines for treating individuals of a similar condition. When information is given to the patient, the information should be comprehensive and correct. This will enable them to make an informed choice. e.g. the therapist has a patient with a lower lumbar complete spinal cord injury. When offering choices, she is bound by the principle of distributive justice, to offer to this patient options of wheelchair as well as ambulation as means of locomotion. However, to respect his autonomy, the therapist is also bound to inform him about the potential benefits of each, the potential costs in time and money including those of long term care. This information should be given to all patients of a similar affectation. It would be unethical to withhold information based on the therapist's assessment of say the patient's financial condition or mental abilities (without objective information stating that he may have poor mentation).

Respect for autonomy also requires us not to deceive, by withholding information or giving false information. Respect for autonomy requires us to be available- be present on time for appointments, communicate well including listening. Respect for autonomy also means that we do not coerce or imply negative results due to non-acquiesance, but rather that we give clear and un-emotional information. e.g. it would be unethical to tell a patient" *if you do not listen to me and walk right now, I am not going to see you again.*" Or "*if you do not do what I say, you are going to be bed-bound for the rest of your life*". These phrases have an undertone of threat even if what the therapist said may be true in the second case.

Respect for autonomy involves an underlying amount of trust. This includes trust in the patient's judgement and the right to make that judgement as well as the patient's trust in the therapist. Respecting the patient's autonomy automatically implies that thc patient and therapist are on the same footing and see each other as equals. In order for the patient to exercise his right to autonomy, this is essential. Fortunately, it is much easier for physiotherapists to gain this mutual trust again due to the nature of care offered by them, in most instances except perhaps ICU care.

How should the therapist interpret autonomy?
To cite an example the therapist has a patient who is fully conscious and is on a ventilator. The patient is unable to speak, but indicates that he does not want to be suctioned. Under the principle of beneficence, the therapist is bound to offer this service as she knows that it is an essential part of care. However the patient's wish is clear. What does the therapist do?

The therapist can explain the benefits of the action and the harm that may entail from withholding it. If the patient still insists and the therapist knows his prognosis is fair-good, the principle of beneficence should take precedence. The therapist must however explain to the patient, and his family why she has to do what she has to do. However if the therapist knows that the prognosis is questionable, and the patient's wishes are clear, the situation leads to a moral dilemma. Perhaps the principle of autonomy should take precedence.

One of the methods to overcome these situations and protect the care providers is the constitution of a "living will". Many countries are increasingly allowing this. What this constitutes, is that an individual, while in good physical and mental health, draws up a legal document which outlines his/her wishes regarding care during situations where he/she may be unable to make his/her wishes clear. But there is a drawback here as well. Most living wills will specify that the document is to be adhered to based on the judgement of the treating physician. A living will can specify the components of terminal care that an individual wishes to be administered. For example, he may wish to have pain medication but no other care. Or he may wish only for oxygen and hydration and no other care. He may wish not to be resuscitated.

Why is autonomy necessary?
The right to autonomy is an essential part of medical ethics due in part to prevent the abuse of position by healthcare practitioners. A case in point would be- with commercial medicine being a reality, nursing homes in provincial India find it necessary to maintain a no or low record of death rates in order to stay afloat. In order to achieve this, it is not uncommon to have patients on life support for no medical reason whatsoever. This scenario may also be repeated by individuals for their own record.

While there is seldom any such motivation for physiotherapists and the circumstances where patients undergoing physiotherapy, exercise their right of autonomy are less dramatic, it is nevertheless an essential part of PT practice as well. Most often except in cases as outlined earlier, the questions would be cessation of treatment, a cheaper treatment option or an alternative treatment as prescribed by the doctor or as experienced earlier by the patient.

What does a breach of autonomy mean?
One of the major areas of autonomy, comes when giving CPR to a patient. As health providers, each of us has a high chance of being in a situation of finding a patient in need of CPR at some point in our careers. If the patient has clearly stated that he does not wish to be resuscitated, this life saving act constitutes a breach of autonomy.

Right to information

What does it mean in the patient-therapist relationship?

While the right to information is essentially a part of "autonomy", there are other aspects to it. A patient who requests specific information on physiotherapeutic treatment options would be fairly easy to handle. However the problem arises when the referring physician has indicated certain treatment modalities, which may be contraindicated or not optimum. The best course of action in such a case is to defer to the senior therapist who should have a working relationship with the physician. When a recommended treatment is changed this should be informed to the patient. Obviously this is best done with the knowledge of the physician. Occasionally, there are instances of unpleasantness which are most often lack of communication between professionals. However it is to be emphasized, that when there is a treatment that is potentially harmful or a substitute that is better, the patient must be given the treatment that the therapist deems best. It would be unethical and an offence if the therapist gives a treatment modality that she knows is harmful in order to defer to the physician. With the present scenario of the absence of a regulatory body for physiotherapists in India, the burden of litigation falls on the physician. Hence it is doubly important in respect to inter-professional ethical conduct, to keep the referring physician informed.

Other aspects of information include, the explanation of potential harm or lack of benefit. Fortunately, there are few if any such situations in physiotherapy. When there are potentially harmful treatment options, substitution with a harmless modality should be instituted and the reasons explained to the patient. An example would be that of the young lady who was given SWD to the low back in the example given earlier. Substitution with a superficial heating modality or exercises or ergonomics would have been the best option. Another minor but important detail is the right of the patient to know the identity of the therapist. This includes name and job position. Name tags must display this prominently.

Why is information necessary?
Knowledge of situations affecting him is the inalienable right of any individual. This holds true in physiotherapeutic treatment as well. Besides this sharing of knowledge with the patient gains his trust. Trust in turn ensures greater cooperation which is essential for the benefits of physiotherapy treatments.

What does a breach of this right mean?
Withholding of information from the patient is a culpable offence if there is litigation. At the least it can constitute a breach of trust and decreased patient participation.

How much information is good enough?

Often there is a conflict of the principles of beneficence and autonomy when it comes to the question of information. Thomas Percival in the nineteenth century, stressed the need to give only so much information as is necessary as too much information especially if it is negative may affect the patient's morale. Is this tenet still valid in today's world when information can be got from a number of sources and often can be misleading? Probably, the best recourse is to answer all direct questions honestly and not volunteer negative information unless that information has a direct impact on the patient's treatment plan.

Dealing with grief

Concomitant with information comes the natural emotion of grief or despair. This is obviously so in the case of chronic disability. How does the therapist deal with this grief? If this reaction comes in the way of the patient's well being or participation with treatment, they must be referred to the appropriate professional. Otherwise, dealing with the person empathetically and pointing out avenues for the future may assist the patient to divert his grief to productive work. This is especially necessary when you are called upon to break the news of permanent disability to a patient.

Another aspect to remember is that as a therapist those individuals under your care are in a vulnerable state of mind. Hence, empathy while dealing with them is absolutely essential.

Respect for the individual

This also falls broadly under the principle of "autonomy". It is unfortunate that even the most well meaning therapist is often found describing her patients as "diseases". For example "that knee arthroplasty in bed number 45". This kind of description dehumanizes the patient and is disrespectful. Another often seen practice is that of health providers talking over a patient, as if he were incapable of following what was being said. This is disrespectful conduct as well.

What does it mean in the patient-therapist relationship? In any kind of treatment, it is essential that the patient is an equal partner. This may be much more so in physiotherapy. This kind of mutual trust and participation cannot be gained unless the therapist treats the patient on an equal footing. This involves respect and the establishment of a relationship based on trust and information.

Restraints

One of the issues here would concern restraining a cognitively impaired individual. It is a common practice, to restrain a restless, violent, a person with poor balance or otherwise hard-to-handle individual. While this is a dehumanizing and disrespectful practice, it is often justified for the person's safety or often for his life itself as in the case of a person who repeatedly extubates himself unless his hands are restrained. However there are certain rules of behaviour that must be adhered to while administering restraints. As chemical (drug) restraints are not within our purview, they will not be considered here. **Physical restraints are mechanisms wherein the individuals ability to move a part of the limb, the whole limb or the whole body is curtailed by means of a physical obstruction.** These consist of straps used for tying a person's hands or legs, mittens, chest straps, pelvic straps, mechanisms in a wheelchair to prevent mobility, locking of doors and windows etc. The rules to be followed in this case are as follows

- Restrain **only** when necessary
- If limbs are restrained, the part must be moved through full ROM at least once every 30 minutes. If the whole person is restrained, he must be allowed to stretch or walk at least every hour.
- The least amount of restraint must be used
- Restraints must be constructed in such a way that applying them will not injure the patient. Care must be taken that there is no injury even with straining.
- A person must be restrained only for the least amount of time that it is essential

- If possible, it is better to have human supervision rather than physical restraints
- The need for the restraint must be explained to the patient/ relatives
- Restraints must **never** be used for the convenience of a therapist or as a mode of punishment.

Gender/culture/age Sensitivity

With globalization, therapists in India may come into contact with patients from different cultures with very different concepts of moral issues. So it is essential that the physiotherapist make a concerted effort to seek information and understand issues of cultural differences as concerns patient under her care.

Consider these simple situations:

Addressing an older person by his first name is considered disrespectful and degrading in most eastern cultures. However this is perfectly natural in western cultures- in fact it is considered friendly.

Likewise when treating a lady, a male therapist should be sensitive enough to have another lady present if it is not possible to have a lady therapist see the patient.

The converse may be true too. For instance many Buddhist monks are averse to a lady touching them and may request a male therapist.

It is necessary for the therapist to be able to accept these situations and take it in her stride and conform to the patients' wishes. Being offended at these situations is unnecessary and counter productive.

What does it mean in the patient-therapist relationship? There are aspects of physiotherapy treatment which may be alien to the culture. This comes into focus often when we advice patients on home modifications or behaviour modification techniques.

Let us consider this example.

A very devout Muslim gentleman undergoes bilateral total knee replacements for severe arthritis. After the surgery the therapist tells him he should not kneel anymore and will be unable to bend his knees more than 90 degrees. This means he will be unable to perform his daily prayers in the prescribed way. The patient is livid. He says that if this information had been told to him prior to surgery, he would never have undergone the surgery.

The pre-op information booklet given to all patients, broadly describes precautions but is not clear about the position of prayer adopted by Muslims. In a country like ours, this cultural insensitivity amounts to a breach of the " right to information" part of the principle of autonomy. One of the ways to help this patient at this juncture would be to suggest that it was very likely that Islam allowed other options if the prescribed manner was not possible and that the patient should consult his religious leaders.

Physiotherapists routinely tell patients to adopt different lifestyles after certain injuries or surgeries without thinking about the cultural implications. It is extremely important to describe in detail, aspects of activities of daily living which may have to undergo change. Suitable alternatives can only be worked out after discussion with the patient to ascertain what is acceptable to him. Enforcing what the therapist thinks is optimum without discussion is a breach of autonomy. This can be a great challenge for the community therapist.

Another important issue is one of age. Someone once said " you may be biased against people because they are a different colour/ religion or gender. But remember if you are prejudiced against someone because of age, you will be in their shoes sooner or later." It might be good to remember this adage. It is unfortunately all too common for therapists to decrease the effort of therapy or the duration or the components just because the patient is in her opinion "too old for that". Who decides this? Not the therapist. It is the prerogative of the patient to decide if he is too old or not old enough. The duty of the therapist is to assess the patient without prejudice and based on the evaluation and the patient's wishes and needs prescribe and give treatment. Of course physiological considerations of age must be kept in mind.

Literature shows that even people in the tenth decade of life can improve strength and fitness with exercises.

Barriers

Barriers are components of the environment that prevent the individual's optimum performance.

Barriers can be socio-cultural, economic, physical, psychological, language etc.

Of these we have dealt with gender and cultural issues. We will now deal with language, economic and psychological barriers.

What does it mean in the patient-therapist relationship? Language barriers are critical in a profession like physiotherapy where there is a great deal of verbal interaction. In a country like India, this means that the therapist must take a great deal of effort while dealing with the patient. Inadequate communication can mean discomfort, and misunderstanding. Every physiotherapy procedure when taught in the classroom stresses on "instruction to the patient". This crucial step is often missed when the lessons are carried over to the clinic. Let us consider the following example.

A patient has been in an accident and has been immobilized for six weeks. Now physiotherapy has been requested. The therapist goes to the patient and without preamble, makes the patient sit up. No one has taken the trouble to explain to the patient, that his period of immobilization is over and he can start to walk. This may be due to the fact that there is no one there who can speak the language. However that does not excuse the incident.

When the therapist attempts to sit the patient up, he resists, he is confused, he may be angry etc. All of these are valid reactions. The therapist has infringed on his right to information and his autonomy.

Another aspect of communication barriers is when the patient or family member, perceive the therapist's best intentions as coercion. One of the necessary evils of physiotherapy as a profession, is that it often involves exercises that cause pain or discomfort. Care must be taken that an unwilling patient is not threatened or coerced but only cajoled and encouraged.

Likewise, there may be treatments that the patient is unwilling to undergo. He may tell the therapist that he can walk with his family members or do the exercises on his own. Often this is inadequate and the therapist's skilled services are required. It is important that the therapist probe the reasons behind his refusal. Is it due to economic concerns? If so is there anything the therapist can do? Very often when working in a hospital, it is not possible for an individual staff member to waive charges of services. In this case, the therapist must consider the option of instructing the family members in continuing the treatment if possible with supervision at intervals. If there are electrical modalities involved or skilled services that are crucial to recovery, the patient's economic concerns must be relayed to administrative authorities and any benefits possible availed of.

The same scenario may present itself if the patient is uncomfortable with the therapist for any reason whatsoever. If this is so, the therapist must make arrangements for someone else to take over immediately without prejudice. The reasons for the patient's discomfort with his therapist may be unimportant and need not be probed unless there is wrong doing on the part of the therapist. Similarly, as mentioned earlier, if the therapist is uncomfortable working with a particular patient, she must make arrangements for an alternate therapist to take over the patient again without prejudice. Another aspect is the use of coercion overt or covert. No form of coercion may be used in a therapist-patient relationship.

Good Samaritan or Good faith rule

This rule pertains to the act of doing the best under the circumstances without thought of future ramifications.

An example of a Good Samaritan is a person who offers first aid or takes an accident victim to a hospital. Most countries have laws that give immunity to such individuals, when their actions may have adverse results or is in conflict with the patient's living will. This can hold good in hospital situations as well. If a patient appears to be in need of resuscitation and a staff member who is unfamiliar with the patient, administers CPR, which is in conflict with the patient's wishes, the staff would be protected from prosecution by this rule. This is because the staff member did not deliberately choose to thwart the patient's right of autonomy, rather she did what was most appropriate under the circumstances. Here the principle of beneficence and justice take precedence.

Why is it necessary?
This rule is necessary as aspects of care falling under this rule are immediate and life saving procedures when seeking information would waste time and risk the patient's life. The immunity granted by law is essential so that health providers do not hesitate to act immediately due to concerns of prosecution.

Unpleasant facts

There are often factors of care or prognosis that may not entirely be the purview of the physiotherapist. However the therapist is often asked questions pertaining to care and prognosis. These questions are often best answered in a team conference. However this only happens at best in rehabilitation centers. If the therapist has inadequate knowledge to answer the questions posed, it is best to be honest about this and tell the patient that the questions may be asked to the physician. The therapist can often aid this discussion by informing the physician about the patient's concerns. Sometimes, the patient may not have understood the medical jargon and may ask for an explanation. This should be given. The earlier example of the child with cerebral palsy illustrates this point.

Legal Issues

Although, there are few cases of litigation against physiotherapists in India, due in large to the absence of a regulatory body and a clear job description, this is not the case elsewhere. Breaches in these issues can lead to litigation. In India, at present it can lead to the patients losing faith in the therapist and may soon lead to litigation.

Professional Conduct

Aspects of professional conduct have an indirect bearing on ethics. This is based on the principles of beneficence and distributive justice. It is extremely important to behave in a professional, unbiased and uniform manner with all patients under one's care. The mantra to be adopted here is "be friendly but not familiar". The amount of time spent with each patient should be based on needs and not because he speaks the same language or is fun to be with or is good looking or any such personal reasons. Aspects of professional behaviour include the following:

Dress: The therapist must dress in a professional manner. This ensures the safety of both therapist and patient. Most institutions have dress codes which ensure this. As mentioned earlier, a therapist who is gait training a patient is responsible to ensure her own safety first. Only if she is comfortable and safe can she perform her job in a safe and responsible manner. For this it is important for instance that she have footwear that is non slippery and gives her the stability she needs.

Language: As stressed earlier, the therapist must attempt to be able to communicate with her patient effectively, either directly or through an interpreter.

Interpersonal relations: While a fair amount of joking and bantering goes on in most physiotherapy departments, it is necessary to ensure that this does not interfere with treatment or foster any negative feelings among patients.

Acceptance of gifts: Other than the prescribed fee for services, no gifts of cash or kind should be accepted from patients.

Prejudices: The therapist must ensure that any personal prejudices she may have with regard to region, religion, language or gender does not come in the way of her treatment and interaction with her patients. If it does, she must hand over the concerned patient to another therapist.

Privacy: The patient's privacy must be ensured. If a particular patient is uncomfortable working in a large gym with other patients, he must be moved to an environment where he is comfortable. Likewise, a lady patient who is uncomfortable with a male therapist must be provided with a female therapist, or if this is impossible, a lady must be in attendance during treatment.

Summary

Thus clinical practice guidelines of ethical conduct fall under the four principles of Beneficence: This principle defines the duty of the health provider to practice in a way that benefits the patient or client under her care.

Autonomy: This principle defines the right of the patient to choose the treatment offered to him and includes his right to refuse any treatment option he may consider as useless or harmful or otherwise.

Distributive justice: This principle defines the distribution of resources in a fair and just manner. In this context, it is generally agreed that "the preferential option for the poor" is justified.

Non-maleficence: This principle defines the duty of the therapist to do no harm.

Additional tenets include:

Confidentiality.

Right to make informed choices.

Right to information.

Respect for the individual.

Gender/culture/age sensitivity.

Barriers.

Good Samaritan rule.

Legal issues.

Professional conduct.

Chapter five

Private Practice

On a personal level, everyone must answer the following question: what is my highest aspiration? The answer might be wealth, fame knowledge, popularity or integrity. But if integrity is secondary to any of the alternatives, it will be sacrificed in situations where a choice must be made. Such situations will inevitably occur in every person's life.
- Murphy Smith

Although patient care whether at a large hospital or in a private clinic would be governed by the same rules of ethical conduct, there are certain additional considerations when one is practicing out of one's own clinic. Quite obviously, there is a definite economic consideration. Any private practice is a business venture and all businesses must make a profit to be viable. The other aspect is as the bulk of physiotherapy practice is rooted in physician referrals, there are social obligations as well. Besides this, it is unethical to engage in business practices unfair to the rest of the profession. We shall deal with some of these issues in this chapter.

Monetary Compensation

The Indian Association of Physiotherapists' guidelines state that the charges for services must be in keeping with the trend in the area of practice. Since there is not and never can be absolute rules of charges for services, these are decided upon based on the geographical location, general economic status, education levels of the population, charges in the same area or neighbouring areas and the possible clientele. We shall take each of these separately.

Geographical location is important in that, costs for all services are generally greater in urban areas than rural. This would hold good for physiotherapy services as well. Exceptions would be in communities that cater to retired populations, upscale holiday environments and areas that are essentially meant for health, or recreation e.g. spas, ski resorts etc. In any area that has more than one business of the same type, there exists either a formal or a tenuous association that would regulate these issues. If this is not the case, the best option is to adopt the guidelines of a similar community. What are the ethical aspects of this? In any area, where there is more than one private physiotherapy clinic, it would be unethical to charge more than or less than one's peers. More than because there is an implication that somehow your services are superior and less than because you are likely to attract more clients and possibly take away clients from your colleagues in the area. The first instance would be unethical practice both to the patient as well as your professional colleagues whereas the second would be unethical to your colleagues. Now what about if you are the only practicing therapist in the area? This would put a greater moral burden while deciding charges for services as you have no one to compare to. There are business implications as well. If you start the practice with low charges and then increase the charges, chances are your reputation and your business will suffer.

Economic status of the general population is of great importance in this case. If the average patient who is likely to seek the services of a therapist is of the working class, the morally right thing would be to charge at the lower end of the spectrum perhaps with packages or other benefits for the economically backward. If the average client is economically well to do, charges can be commensurate with what is optimum.

Education levels of the population that you are catering to is important. The educated and aware individuals are likely to be more inquisitive about their treatment details and more likely to demand value for money in that you may be expected to prognosticate the number of visits they are likely to need to take care of a certain problem and more likely to compare costs of other therapists in the area etc. The therapist has a greater moral responsibility when the education and awareness level of her clientele is low. In this situation, she has to take cognisance of the value for money and prognostic aspects and choose her charging system carefully.

The other aspect to take into consideration is the kind of patients one is likely to encounter. Are there any diseases or dysfunction, which are endemic to the particular area? Are there a lot of chronically disabled individuals? Are patients likely to return time after time? If for instance there is a large employer from whom you are likely to get substantial number of patients, it would be worthwhile to work out some sort of employee health benefit scheme with the administration of the company, rather than charge patients on a per visit system. The same kind of system can be tailored to individuals as well.

The next issue that is of importance in private practice that we shall deal with is **treatment duration.** It maybe tempting to increase the duration of a treatment or prolong the number of visits when the patient is willing and there is economic benefit. Obviously this is inappropriate. Often for ease of management, private clinics set charges for a period of time usually 20-30 minutes a session. If the patient can tolerate greater duration and increase in duration would be beneficial to the patient, this would be appropriate so long as the patient understands the financial implications of prolonging treatment. However if benefits are uncertain, this is unethical practice even if the patient is aware, cooperative or even insistent. *For example there is no added benefit to applying SWD for 1 hour as opposed to the generally accepted 15-20 minutes. In fact there are or can be harmful effects. On the other hand, there are definite effects of doing mobilisation exercises for 1 hour as opposed to 20 minutes.*

Unnecessary/inappropriate Treatment

Going hand in hand with prolongation of treatment duration, is the application of unnecessary or inappropriate treatment for economic gain.

A very common scenario in India unfortunately, is the application of electrical stimulation in children with cerebral palsy/ individuals after stroke or head injury etc by private practitioners. Although there is some mention in the literature of beneficial effects of this modality in these patients, often the motivation is merely, to convince the patient and family of some fancy treatment being done. Often these treatments are carried out for months or years.

The other scenario is that of applying treatment modalities on the request of patients/ families/ referring physicians. The therapist wrongly justifies this action by applying vicarious liability to the person who has requested the treatment. However this is not pardonable. As a professional it is your duty to do only those things that you deem beneficial to the patient under your care. The greater moral responsibility lies with you. If the patient is insistent and refuses to see reason, there is no harm in telling him that you will only do what you deem fit and if he is dissatisfied, he can seek another therapist. Seldom is this necessary however. Is it wrong to offer treatment that will have no potential harm but benefit is questionable? If the situation is explained to the patient and he understands the lack of benefit but requests that the treatment be done anyway, it is justified as we cannot completely rule out the benefits of placebo therapy. To take the following example:

A patient has been coming to you for non specific back ache. There are no clinical signs. You start out treatment with hot packs followed by exercises. After two days, you tell the patient that purely exercises are enough and he need not come to you anymore. The patient however says that the hot packs give him some temporary relief and he would like to continue coming. You tell him that the hot packs are merely to increase comfort and he can have the same benefit by taking a hot shower at home. The patient is unconvinced and says he would still like to come. You are entirely justified in allowing him to continue for a specific time period and charging him for it.

Taking the same scenario a little further, how does a therapist curtail treatment for an insistent patient? This often becomes a factor especially in the case of malingerers or those who have third party payers like employers. Patients may come seeking or demanding treatment even though in your best clinical judgement they do not require treatment. Like many of the other issues, there is no easy answer. One must take each case on its own merit taking care to maintain professional decorum during all dealings.

Conflict of Interest

This issues comes about when there are incentives to be gained from doing a particular treatment. Although this is far more common where pharmaceutical companies are pushing new drugs, it is feasible that the same scenario may arise when new equipment come into the market. The manufacturer may offer incentives, if you apply the treatment to a number of subjects in order to give an anecdotal advertisement for the product. If this happens the therapist may find her judgement clouded by the attraction of the incentive. This would go against the principle of non-malnce. Another scenario can be envisioned as described below:

There are several private practice clinics in an area. Most of them offer LASER therapy for a variety of ailments. You find that there is inconclusive evidence as to the efficacy of LASER and haven't bothered to buy a machine. Soon you find patients are asking you why you do not have a LASER when all others do. In order to keep your clientele, you might be tempted to join the bandwagon. This again constitutes a condition of conflict of interests.

Referee Fee

Unfortunately, it has come to be the practice, that physicians who refer patients for therapy expect and are given a referee fee. Is this ethical? While that is not within the scope of this book to discuss, we shall consider the practice of giving a referee fee. In this case the therapist who gives a referee fee is as culpable as the physician who takes it. Why is this so? By offering a referee fee, there is an implied temptation for the physician to refer more cases to you. The incentive offered will cloud his clinical judgement and patients who would otherwise not have been referred for physiotherapy may be referred. Likewise as it is a mutually beneficial situation, therapists may find that their clinical judgement in turn is clouded and they tend to treat even those patients who may not require therapy.

Another pitfall in the referee fee system is the temptation to refer your patients only to those professionals who gives you a fee regardless of their competence to manage the particular patient. And quite obviously, the added economic burden falls on the patient.

Staffing

Employment of staff in private clinics is another important issue. As financial viability of the business depends on low overheads, it maybe tempting to staff the clinic with employees who are not qualified as they will demand lesser pay. Another way of decreasing overheads is by employing staff on a temporary basis which precludes the employer from offering benefits. Another tendency is to staff inadequately or have double job descriptions i.e. The same person fulfils two jobs e.g. clerk and attendant. All of these instances are a violation of ethical clinical practice. Staff, especially those who come into direct patient contact, must be suitably qualified. If for instance the clinic takes on interns or students their position must be clearly defined and displayed so that the patient is aware of the presence of student therapists. It is also imperative that name tags are visibly worn. In addition, the rights of the patient under the consumer protection act must be displayed including the contact details of the local forum in case of complaints. Another issue is staff satisfaction. Morale of the employees will reflect on the quality of their work output. This in turn will ensure patient satisfaction. Hence it is important that employee morale is made a priority.

Primary Contact

When the therapist is the primary contact professional, this brings to the fore certain other issues that may have an import on professional ethics.

When the patient comes to the therapist through a physician, the patient is merely indicating his trust in the physician by complying with his advice. Trust in the therapist as a professional must be gained later. When a patient comes directly without a physician's referral, there is an implied trust in the therapist herself. This trust must be nurtured through appropriate practice guidelines. First and foremost, if the problems that the patient presents with are beyond the scope of physiotherapy or may lead to other complications at a later date, the patient **MUST** be referred to the appropriate medical doctor. This referral must be done prior to any physiotherapy intervention. The next issue comes to referee fee. As mentioned earlier, it is unethical to offer or take referee fees. With relevance to physiotherapists; this includes occupational therapists, physicians, orthotics and prosthetic professionals and medical equipment dealers. As already explained earlier, a system of referee fee will result in a conflict of interests and the best interests of the patient will not be served.

Non Patient Clientele

With physiotherapists becoming increasingly involved in preventive aspects of health rather than actual patient care, the number of clients who are not patients is rapidly increasing. This population unlike the patient population is obviously less vulnerable and more likely to seek evidence and options for therapy. The relationship tends to be more on an equal footing. This involves therapists who are running health clubs, fitness programmes or sport rehabilitation. While the four principles of ethics remain relevant, the relationship here is more likely based on equality rather than in a patient-therapist relationship. Here the onus shifts from the client to the therapist.

Location and Building

There is also the consideration of location and building safety. If the clinic is situated in an area that is exposed to noxious effluents or has unsafe water supply or other safety and health issues, the therapist owning the building may have a certain amount of vicarious responsibility. Likewise a building which is unsafe or inaccessible could also prove a liability. If the therapist does not have the luxury of relocating, she must at least take the precaution of posting signs that would make her clientele aware of the potential hazards if any. Pure unpleasantness without any known health hazards need not be emphasised. However if long term exposure may cause deleterious effects, the employees must be made aware. For example a clinic situated near a busy railway track may cause health hazards from long term exposure to the vibration and sound. However short term effects are negligible. In this case only the employees need to be made aware of the situation and not the patients. An inaccessible building must have provision for easy transfer of patients. This depends on the type of patients who normally visit the clinic. If the clinic caters to individuals who come for fitness reasons alone a clinic on the first floor without lift facilities is perfectly acceptable. If however the clinic also sees patients who are patients, this is not acceptable.

Another consideration is ease of evacuation in case of natural disasters. It is essential for the clinic to have recognised routes of evacuation in case of varying natural disasters like fire, earthquake and flood. All staff must be well versed with the procedure to be followed in case of disaster. These are responsibilities, whose non compliance can lead to litigation.

Summary

Issues that affect the private practitioner are as follows:

Fixing charges for services.

Treatment duration, type, indications, cessation

Staffing appropriately.

Referee fee.

Conflict of interest.

Primary contact.

Normal clientele.

Vicarious responsibility pertaining to location and building.

Chapter six

Issues in Academics

To educate a person in mind and not in morals is to educate a menace to society.
—Theodore Roosevelt

So far we have dealt with responsibilities towards patients which is the primary and most far reaching part of ethical practice. We shall now deal with issues of academics with regard to physiotherapy education in India.

Academic Integrity

Integrity involves firm adherence to academic honesty and to ethical conduct consistent with values based on standards that respect the intellectual efforts of both oneself and others. The five values that are most important are honesty, integrity, respect, accountability and academic responsibility. We shall see what each of these values means in different contexts and to different individuals.

Students

Academic integrity in relation to the student consists of not cheating, being on time for classes, completing assignments thoroughly and on time, giving feedback to teachers with honesty and in an unbiased manner, not misrepresenting or misquoting sources, behaving always in a professional and dignified manner, being courageous enough to offer constructive criticism to peers and faculty, and exposing unethical behaviour. For example not giving information that a student is not sure of about a patient, or information that he thinks may invite criticism is one way of cheating. Taking information from medical files when the expectation is that the student arrives at this information on his own is another form of cheating. Standards of academic honesty are violated whenever a student engages in any action that jeopardizes the integrity of scholarly work. Such actions include cheating in the classroom or on examinations, including clinical examinations; the intentional and deliberate misuse of data in order to draw conclusions that may not be warranted by the evidence; fabrication of data; omission or concealment of conflicting data for the purpose of misleading other scholars; use of another's words, ideas, or creative productions without citation in either the text or in footnotes; paraphrasing or summarizing another's material in such a way as to misrepresent the author's intentions; and use of privileged material or unpublished work without permission. Academic dishonesty is a serious matter for professional students committed to intellectual pursuits, and it should be adjudicated strictly and unbiasedly.

Faculty

As a teacher, the faculty member has the responsibility for creating in her classroom or laboratory a climate that encourages the student to learn. The faculty member should exemplify high scholarly standards and respect and foster the student's educational goals.

The faculty member must make clear the objectives of the course or program, establish requirements, set standards of achievement, and evaluate the student's performance in an unbiased and fair manner. The faculty have the responsibility to meet classes as scheduled and, when circumstances prevent this, to ensure that information is conveyed to the student. In addition it is her responsibility to ensure missed classes are made up without undue inconvenience to students.

The faculty member has the responsibility to teach courses in a manner that is consistent with the course description and with the announced objectives of the course. He or she must not intentionally interject into classes material or personal views that have no pedagogical relationship to the subject matter of the course. The content of classes must be current and in keeping with the level of knowledge expected of the students. On controversial issues within the scope of the course a reasonable range of opinion should be presented. When the faculty member presents his or her own views on such issues, they should always be identified as such. Wherever values, judgments, or speculative opinions constitute part of the subject matter, they should be identified as such and should not be offered as fact.

The faculty member has a responsibility to ensure a fair and impartial evaluation of the student's work. Such evaluation should be consistent with recognized standards and must not be influenced by irrelevancies such as religion, race, sex, or political views, or be based on the student's agreement with the teacher's opinion pertaining to matters of controversy within the discipline.

Every student is entitled to the same intellectual freedom which the faculty member enjoys. The faculty member must respect that freedom. Restraint must not be imposed upon the student's search for or consideration of diverse or contrary opinion. More positively, the faculty member has an obligation to protect the student's freedom to learn. When the students present an opposing view on controversial topics, that view must be discussed with the same gravity as other views. It is not always the case that the teacher knows best!

The classroom must remain a place where free and open discussion of all content and issues relevant to a course can take place.

The faculty member has obligations as an intellectual guide and counselor to students. He or she has a responsibility to be available to students for private conferences. In advising students, every reasonable effort should be made to see that information given to them is accurate.

he should always respect the confidence deriving from the faculty-student relationship.

The faculty member must avoid exploitation of students for personal advantage. For example, in writings and oral presentations due acknowledgment of their contributions to the work should be made.

Faculty also have to demonstrate integrity in their dealing with their superiors. It is important to adhere to department or college policies and any lack of agreement among faculty must not be visible to students. This will undermine the sanctity of the education process. Policies of the university must be understood and adhered to. This does not mean that she must follow them without question. Integrity also means that she have the courage to question or challenge those policies that may be lacking in integrity.

Administrators

It is the responsibility of administrators to ensure availability of an atmosphere conducive to learning. This involves staffing adequately, showing appreciation for work done, promoting a friendly and convivial environment, providing for adequate infrastructure, addressing student and faculty grievances honestly and sincerely, defining responsibilities of faculty, having clear rules and enforcing them consistently and all together upholding the values described above.

Ensuring integrity in academic work is a joint enterprise involving both faculty and students. Among the most important goals of professional education are maintaining an environment of academic integrity and instilling in students a lifelong commitment to the academic honesty that is fundamental to good scholarship. These goals are best achieved as a result of effective dialogue between students and faculty mentors regarding academic integrity and by the examples of members of the academic community whose intellectual accomplishments demonstrate sensitivity to the nuances of ethical conduct in scholarly work.

The basic functions of a university are the advancement and dissemination of knowledge, the development of critical intelligence, and the education of citizens and professional workers for the society of which the university is a part. The indispensable condition for the successful discharge of these functions is an atmosphere of intellectual freedom. Unless he or she is free to pursue the quest for knowledge and understanding, wherever it may lead, and to report and discuss the findings, whatever they may be, the faculty member cannot properly perform his or her work. As a participant in an enterprise that depends upon freedom for its health and integrity, the faculty member has a special interest in promoting conditions of free inquiry and furthering public understanding of academic freedom. Freedom entails responsibilities. It is incumbent upon the faculty member to accept the responsibilities which are concomitant with the freedom he or she needs. Those responsibilities are (1) to students, (2) to the profession (3) to colleagues, (4) to the university, and (5) to the larger community which the university serves. To make these responsibilities operational, it is necessary that ethical and professional standards be adopted to guide faculty members in their conduct and that effective mechanisms be established to monitor and enforce compliance with these standards. Responsibilities to students and the university have been outlined in the previous section. We shall take a look at the other responsibilities now.

Responsibilities to Colleagues

As a colleague, the faculty member has obligations that derive from common membership in the profession. She must respect and defend the free inquiry of associates and avoids interference with their work. In the exchange of criticism and ideas, she must show due respect for the rights of others to their opinions. She must refrain from personal vilification and acknowledge contributions of others to her work. When asked to evaluate the professional performance of a colleague, the faculty member must strive to be objective.

Responsibilities to the Profession

As an academician, it is the duty of the faculty to ensure advancement of the profession she subscribes to. This involves, engaging in research, dissipation of knowledge gained from research, keeping up-to-date with professional growth, ensuring membership in professional bodies and adhering to their norms, promoting professional growth of self and colleagues, and ensuring that no action of hers can be detrimental to the profession.

Responsibilities to the Community

As a physiotherapist, the academician must ensure that her increased knowledge serves the community at large. This can involve newspaper articles, public awareness programes aimed at both prospective therapists and patients private dialogue etc. It is also an important aspect to ensure that no adverse or wrong information is dissipated. If perchance such a lapse occurs, it is the moral responsibility of the person to correct her mistake at the earliest in a thorough manner. It is pertinent to note that all actions of an academician have a far reaching effect on the community due to the simple fact that a large number of students are influenced by her. At all times the academician must be a role model for her students, colleagues, and the community.

There has been a boom in the number of colleges offering undergraduate and more recently post-graduate education in India since the 1990s. Due to this "explosion of education" as it were, it is necessary to look at some of the practices of these institutions. As was pointed out in the chapter on private clinics, education institutions especially those run by private houses are obviously business concerns. Here the student is the consumer and in that capacity has certain expectations and rights. Conversely the institution and the faculty have certain duties and responsibilities towards the student and the profession at large. The following section will take a look at these issues.

Inadequate knowledge of profession of the administrators

It is disheartening to note that many of the administrative heads of educational institutions launch the course of physiotherapy along with such unlikely other courses as fashion design and catering. This scenario is due to the fact that courses are launched with only the financial objective in mind. This leads to colleges functioning without basic infrastructural requirements of building space, basic sciences laboratories and faculty, adequate core faculty and very often even without a hospital affiliation. Perhaps what is even more disheartening is that these colleges continue to function in sub standard conditions with full strength. This points to total disregard for the profession, the patients who are the end beneficiaries and the students' future career prospects. It is not inconceivable that in the near future, such institutions may be held liable for the negligent practice by their students who may claim inadequate education. The responsibility of administrators is that they make an effort to understand the requirements and implications of the courses that they propose to launch and make a sincere effort to meet these requirements. The profit motive must be curbed for the initial few years.

Advertisement

In many countries it is essential for a student applying to physiotherapy schools to show proof of volunteer hours. This means that the student has actually worked in a volunteer capacity in a variety of physiotherapy departments and knows what the profession entails. This is an excellent admission requirement. But as the education system in India propels the student to make a career choice very early in life, this system becomes inapplicable here. Due to this, the student often has no inkling of what the profession she is seeking admission for consists of. It is rarely the student who makes the career choice rather it is the parents. This makes it imperative for advertising to be clear, informative and conclusive. Practically speaking what most parents are looking for in the choice of a career for their children is the earning capacity of the profession. Unfortunately, this cannot be predicted as it is a supply-demand dilemma. But advertisements often make the most of this aspect by promising jobs overseas etc. The terminology is such that the promise is implied and hence there is no real responsibility. A responsible and ethical advertisement (the course prospectus) would have the following aspects:

- Objective of the course
- Actual working environment details with examples.
- Average pay after completion of the course at that point in time in different geographical areas
- Prospects for further education
- Pictures of therapists in actual work situations.
- Contact details of faculty for clarification of doubts.

Admission Process

The next issue is that of the actual admission process. During this juncture, the student and her family are in the final decision making process. They may have various options in hand and have to find a clincher. It would be good procedure at this time to give them a tour of the facilities of the college and ensure that the student understands what she is opting for. Students and families may request information on past students and how the institution ranks in the country. Having this information is essential so that there is no urge to gloss over the truth or make vague statements.

Fee structure—hidden Fees

Coming to the financial aspects, fees, like charges for clinical services must be fixed based on general consensus between colleges in the area. Minor variations are justified as the facilities in each college will vary to some extent. But what are most important from the ethical point of view are hidden fees or fees levied for facilities that do not exist or fees levied for essential parts of the course. Hidden fees are capitation fees or fees that are not mentioned in any of the documents until admission process is complete. Fees levied for facilities that do not exist are an all too common scenario. Library fees where there are no libraries and computer lab fees where there are no computers are a regular feature. The other sort of unethical fee levy is fees some institutions charge for hospital facilities. Hospital visits are part of the established curriculum of physiotherapy education in this country and hence any hospital charges that the institution incurs must be borne by the institution itself.

Faculty Student Ratio

A reasonable student to teacher ratio must be maintained consistently. IAP guidelines stipulate the number of faculty of various designations required for conducting the course. These guidelines are very reasonable and must be adhered to. What is the reasoning behind these ratios? As physiotherapy is a hands on profession it entails an inordinate amount of skills. These skills cannot be learnt unless there is on-site supervision both during practice sessions and during clinical work. Hence a small student-teacher ratio is essential for ensuring competency of the students. Having less than necessary faculty would mean that the education imparted to students is not up to par. This is irresponsible and not giving value-for money. In order to get around the IAP regulations the course of action followed by many institutions is to co-opt faculty from other institutions and put their names on the college rolls during IAP inspection. What is noteworthy here is that several academicians are willing to participate in this farce. Both the institution which encourages this practice and the faculty who are willing to participate are engaging in unethical practice. Since there is no statutory regulating professional body in India, these instances go on without disciplinary action being taken.

Depth of Instruction

Coming to actual learning outcomes, there needs to be clearly defined norms of content for each subject taught in the curriculum. This is necessary for many reasons. As there is no licensing system for physiotherapists in India, the burden of proof falls on the university to which the student is affiliated to. Often the syllabus committees of these universities do not have adequate representation from physiotherapy academicians. Even when they do, updating of syllabi is done infrequently and haphazardly. So it falls on the individual college to ensure that adequate knowledge is imparted to students.

Subject matter can be broadly divided as "need to know", "good to know" and "nice to know". The first category is essential knowledge or minimum information that a student **MUST** possess to complete the particular course. The second category consists of information that is very useful and frequently necessary. The last category consists of information that has very little direct impact on routine work but is more of academic interest. When defining the depth of instruction of a particular topic, these points must be kept in mind. The first category must be emphasized on and **ALL** students must have thorough knowledge of it. The second category should also be emphasized and **ALL** students must have at least **rudimentary** knowledge of it. The third category need not be emphasized but must be mentioned and undue weightage must not be given in the student's understanding of these concepts. It is important to ensure that these categories are clearly defined from time to time as knowledge is dynamic. Care must be taken to define ultimate objectives and only then can knowledge depth be defined.

Overlap into other Areas

No discipline in medicine stands alone. This is obvious as no system in the human body can function alone. Since there is a great deal of overlap in the various disciplines, it is irrational to draw imaginary lines of discipline specific areas. For example saying that an occupational therapist must not gait train a patient or use electrical stimulation is impractical because as part of ADL training, an OT would have to assess ambulatory function and she may also use stimulation as a modality to improve muscle power. Likewise a physiotherapist being told not to do a hand assessment or fashion a splint for a patient is also irrational. Especially in a country like India, multidisciplinary rehabilitation teams still remaining a distant dream, these kinds of turf wars are counter productive. Any professional who has pride in her profession will essentially only practice the art and science of that profession. While teaching, this part must be emphasized. Splint making for example would fall into the "nice-to-know" category for an undergraduate student. This is not unethical. However, teaching a physiotherapy student to prescribe medication taken orally or a diet would be unethical due to the possible hazards of such an action without proper knowledge.

Use of Patients for teaching purposes

Physiotherapy education in India differs from its counterpart in the west in that we use real patients for clinical teaching. In western countries which have licensure procedures for physiotherapists, the students handle patients only after successful completion of course work. In India, students start handling patients from the second or third year onwards immediately after they have completed their basic courses. Sometimes the student may not have been successful in anatomy or exercise therapy but would have completed minimum requirements to be promoted to the third year. This is a great risk. Not only are the students unaware of what is to be done in case of untoward instances, they may not even recognize untoward incidents! Going back to the student-teacher ratio, on-site continuous supervision is necessary during all student initiated treatment sessions. Moreover, the patient must be aware that he is being treated by a student and the supervising therapist must be aware that the patient has the right to demand that a therapist see him instead. If this request is made, ethically the therapist must comply gracefully. The other thing that the supervising therapist must ensure is that she does periodic evaluations and modifies the treatment as necessary. This aids learning as well as ensures that the patient does not meet with any detrimental effects due to the student therapist. Often, when students treat patients, charges are waived. But this does not take care of ethical responsibility, but merely ensures that the institution is protected from litigation due to the clause in the consumer protection act which stipulates that if the service is free of charge there is no grounds for litigation. As for the responsibility of the teacher towards the students, care must be taken to ensure that appropriate patients are given to them and the therapist is always available for guidance. This will promote learning as well as ensure that the patient gets appropriate treatment.

Examiner

As at least 50% of the examination procedure consists of a practical and viva voce examination where it is impossible to blind the examiner as to the students' identity, bias either positive or negative is a factor that should be discussed. This bias can come from both the internal and the external examiner. As the student is evidently at the mercy of the examiner and there is no mechanism to ensure what questions are asked etc, examiners are especially responsible for their actions. Other ethical issues in examinations include, bribing the examiner, being unnecessarily emotional to attain sympathy from the examiner, the examiner not really examining the student or asking irrelevant, personal or inappropriate questions, being rude and abusive etc. Universities have certain mechanisms to curb unethical practices among students and examiners. Some of these include the appointment of a third party observer who has no powers to mark the performance but gives a report on the other aspects mentioned above. Other mechanisms are institution of a panel of examiners rather than just one, enforcing detailed documentation of all questions and answers given which is signed by the student as well etc. While these measures are useful, it is essential that both the examiner and the examinee maintain professional decorum and complete the task responsibly.

Specialization

This issue brings to fore the emerging trend in physiotherapy higher education. Any profession that grows eventually has to split into sections or specializations in order to foster growth. Universities recognize this requirement and offer specializations at the post-graduate level. The only issue here is that specializations be offered considering the following:

- Is there a vast enough body of knowledge in the specialty area
- Does the institution have adequate infrastructural facilities and faculty to fulfill the course objectives?

Another important point that specialty faculty must ensure is that there should at no time be any hint of a hierarchy in specialties. For instance there should be no indication on the part of faculty that neurosciences is superior to orthopaedics. Derogatory comments about another specialty must not be made in the hearing of students. Differences in patient care between specialties can be emphasized and one's own inclinations can be put forward as a view point. There is an attitude that is becoming prevalent that ICU therapists are the elite lot due to their work which involves critical patients and therapists working in CBR areas are on the lowermost rung of the ladder due to their not so glamorous working conditions. Any such notions among students must be dispelled by faculty.

Prohibitive Actions

These refer to actions that are in some way an infringement of the rights of another individual. Threats of punitive action in exams, unreasonable attendance requirements, imposing of fines as punishment for lapses like late coming, unreasonable curfew hours in hostels etc would fall into this. Obviously, since they infringe on the basic rights of a individual, they are unethical.

Summary

Issues of academic integrity pervades into all spheres of education like

Student
Faculty
University
Administration
Admission
Instruction
Examination
Punitive action

Chapter seven

Clinical Research

Ethics is in origin the art of recommending to others the sacrifices required for cooperation with oneself
- Bertrand Russell

INTRODUCTION

Ethics in research gained importance in the late 20th century. In the aftermath of World War II, there was an increasing awareness on ethical principles underlying human research. This heightened awareness on ethics for research endeavors was due to the unforgettable inhuman studies, which the medical world witnessed in this era. To name, coerced participation of human captives of Second World War in gruesome research by German scientists, and secondly the syphilis study –withholding the treatment for syphilis patients even after the discovery of penicillin. Such events led to the development of ethical norms and review boards to conserve the human rights in biomedical research.

In the present scenario even those who are victims of fatal illnesses, wanting to be test subjects under experimental conditions, have an ethical review system designed to protect them. These events are leading to an evolution of new norms in ethical research everyday and the developments in the recent years have been tumultuous.

Human Rights in Biomedical Research—A Background

No one shall be subjected to torture or to cruel, inhuman or degrading treatment or punishment. In particular no one shall be subjected without his consent to medical or scientific treatment
-International covenant on civil and political rights

Ethical principles to prevent, researchers abusing human subjects in clinical experimentation have been developing since the Second World War. Many unconscionable studies degrading human rights were brought to the lime light since then. One such was the introduction of cancer cells into elderly patients without their knowledge. Another well-publicised study started in 1930, involved withholding the treatment for syphilis even after the discovery of Penicillin, which extended till 1970's. Following the publicity of this study, the US president apologised and compensated the relatives of the victims.

The Nuremberg code of 1947(Annexure), prevented a repeat of the scenario of war captives used in research by Nazi physicians in the post war era. The Nuremberg code emphasized that the participant should voluntarily consent after getting true information from the researcher about the study, nature of the study, benefits, and potential risks of harm. This code laid the foundations for the currently practiced norm of informed consent. In 1948, the General assembly of United Nations expressed concern for human rights in medical research.

The World Health organization raised concerns in order to develop ethical guidelines, which were in a broader context in the Nuremberg code. In 1964, based on preliminary efforts of the council for organizations of medical sciences, the World Medical association at Helsinki declared certain general principles for use of human subjects in biomedical research. The declaration of Helsinki II (modified in 1975) brought forth many issues which were not addressed until then. These include review of research by the institutional committees. It put forth certain ethical principles, and emphasized that research not conducted according to the mentioned principles should not be accepted for publication. The Helsinki declaration has been modified many times since then.

In 1974, the National Commission for the Protection of Human Subjects of Biomedical and Behavioural Research was commissioned by the National research act, USA (Belmont Report). *The Belmont Report* established three fundamental ethical principles that are relevant to all research involving human subjects: Respect for Persons, Beneficence, and Justice.

The World Health Organization proposed international guidelines for biomedical research involving human subjects in 1982. The guidelines were prepared based on the guidelines for human research put forth by various councils and regulatory bodies in their jurisdictions.

The Indian council of medical research released a policy statement on ethical considerations in research on human subjects in 1980. Later in 2000, ICMR released a statement of '*Ethical Guidelines for Biomedical Research with Human subjects*' which is presently known as ICMR code. ICMR emphasises that all the medical sciences institutes in India conducting research practices should follow the *ICMR Codes*.

Ethical Principles in Biomedical Research involving Humans

Ethical principles put forth in the Belmont report in 1976, apply to all biomedical research with human subjects and well accepted in most cultural traditions. There are three basic principles concerning ethical issues in human research.

Autonomy—refers to the right of each participant as a person to make an informed decision about participation in the study. The investigator must ensure that the participant has received a full disclosure of the nature of the study, the risks, benefits and alternatives, with an extended opportunity to ask questions. The principle of autonomy is ensured with the informed consent taken from the participant by the investigator prior to the study.

Beneficence—refers to the obligation from the investigator to ensure that the participant gains maximum benefits of the study and, to reduce the possible risks of harm to them. A thorough benefit/risk calculation should be done prior to setting the hypothesis to reduce the risks for the participant and/or the society.

The principle of **Justice**—ensures the fair selection of participants, i.e., avoiding participant populations that may be unfairly forced to participate. For example, avoiding prisoners and institutionalized children coerced into participation of research. The investigator should also ensure the equal distribution of benefits and burden on all the participant population groups.

ICMR a regulatory body for research in India has identified twelve principles in guidelines for research using human beings as subjects. The principles put forth by ICMR were found to overlap with other contexts of ethical issues and these are discussed elsewhere in this chapter. The statement of general principles from ICMR (ICMR Code) is attached as an annexure.

Integrity of the Researcher

Research designates an activity designed to test a hypothesis, permit conclusions to be drawn, and thereby to develop or contribute to generalized knowledge. Ethical issues in research include the conduct of the researcher in planning and execution of the research and valuing and protection of the subjects. When a physiotherapist is part of research carried out by a clinician, her conduct should be in keeping with the statuary organization for the profession and as well the ethical guidelines governing the research area. Researchers should maintain high levels of honesty and integrity. A researcher should never condone dishonesty in terms of fraud, falsification and other forms of research falsehood at anytime.

Autonomy in research also refers to the researcher's freedom in selecting meaningful topic of his/her interest, but on the other hand, he/she should have societal and professional responsibilities—in setting the research priorities. Ethical principles dictate a rational development of the theoretical base and sound design in carrying out research.

Research in clinical practice refers to testing interventions that are designed solely to enhance the well-being of an individual patient or client and that have a reasonable expectation of success. This implies that it's unethical to involve patients/clients in research with potential risk of harm and little chance of success and very little to make or add to scientific knowledge.

The researcher must obtain a written, well informed consent from each participant. The participants should be given the right to decide about participation after going through the risks and benefits of the study. Informed consent is an ongoing process and not a singular process or mere formality. When uncertainty exists about the true benefits of intervention the researcher should not bias the participants for inclusion in the study and/or group. For example in a study comparing the effects of two interventions over the disease process, and where there is uncertainty about which is superior researcher should genuinely explain the aspects of both the interventions to the participants.

The researcher should maintain a high level of privacy and confidentiality towards participant's data, and should be sensitive to the issues concerning it. He/she should have worked on, how to communicate to participants in the event of unforeseen findings during the course of the study. In case of any adverse events, how the participants will be managed and dispersal of compensation to the participants should be planned and enumerated.

When it comes to research designs with a control group, it is always a debate among true clinicians, whether to have a control group or not. Having a control group, means this group will receive no treatment or sham treatment. This raises questions of wrong doing, by withholding treatment for the participating population. Due to this concern, present day studies compare the efficacy of one treatment over the other, or the control group will receive the existing conventional treatment or will receive treatment after the study. The last option is only acceptable if delaying treatment will have no adverse effects. For example delaying a treatment modality for three weeks in chronic non specific low back pain will have no adverse effects. However use of a control group is substantiated in certain situations like, when no beneficial treatment exists and/or when the researcher wants to prove the adversity of existing treatment.

The sample size should be of great concern for any research and the size should be decided according to the rationale of the study, the area of research and with the use of statistical methods. During any phase of the study the researcher should control the personal bias and avoid the possible confounding factors which could affect the study results. The researcher should take utmost care to avoid errors in measurements and should use measures of high validity and reliability. In physiotherapy research, there exists a dearth of valid and objective outcome measures. Most of the research studies have reported the use of subjective scales for example ADL score, Functional independence measures (FIM). In such situations use of subjective tools as an outcome measures are accepted subjected to reliability and validity of the tool for the target population. Manipulation of data and inappropriate use of statistical tests to increase the significance of the results for personal benefit are fraudulent.

Appropriate statistical procedure should be used and all observed and measured data should be analyzed and only the true results should be reported. Instances of fraudulent reports do not serve the pursuit of research in the end. The researcher should not suppress or manipulate the results in order to be in conformance with the funding organizations/agents.

Not the least in ethical considerations is authorship. Many instances exist, wherein those who have no or minimal input to the research, insist that their name appear in the research publication. The order/sequence of name quoted in the publication should be determined depending on the amount of work done in the research and or the contribution made by the person(s) in the study and not based on hierarchy. Coercion in this area is also unacceptable.

Informed Consent

The foundations of informed consent in biomedical research were developed in 1947 in Nuremberg as mentioned earlier. The Nuremberg code was the first instance to emphasize that, it is the right of the individual to decide on participation in the research. Informed consent is an indication of the individual giving consent to voluntarily participate in the research after getting true information on research, benefit/risks involved in the study. The various components of informed consent are—disclosure of true information, strategy of management of adverse events, benefits, information regarding confidentiality, compliance of the researcher to answer queries of participants at anytime and the participant's competency and consent.

Components of Informed Consent

Information about the Research

The first part of an informed consent should start with an introduction of the author with invitation to the participant. It should consist of research hypothesis, stating its importance and need in the field. This ensures the participants compliance with the author's idea or belief. The complete procedure of the research should be explained. What will be done, what they will feel during the procedure, how long the procedure will take, duration of the study, what are the benefits, side effects and the potential risks of harm in the procedure to the participants should be explained in the written format. In case of questionnaires, the type of questions asked, how the data would be processed, and confidentiality of the patient data are required. The information should not be deceptive by omission.

In situations, were the researcher believes that the disclosure of information to the participant might affect the results; the institutional review boards may allow the omission in the informed consent. For example, in a study measuring the psychophysical response to exercises, explaining to the subject may lead the participant to overexert himself. This may end in harming the participant or may affect the outcome of the study. However, the participant should be informed about the omission of certain information due the nature of the study, and assured that the complete information will be provided at the end of the study/procedure.

The important aspect of the information is explanation of possible social, psychological or physical risks involved in the procedure. Any foreseeable risk of harm should be informed to the participant. A statement of agreement by the participant about the understanding of the nature of risks should be included. For example, if heat modality is one of the interventions of the study; the participant should be aware of heat boils and burns being the potentials harms in the procedure. In addition, in situations of adverse events how it will be managed, medical care and compensations allowable should be stated. In research involving treatment interventions, participants should be informed about the existence of other modalities and the participant should be given the right to voluntarily participate in the study.

The researcher without any deception or delineation should inform the participant about the benefits for the participant volunteering for the study. The statement should detail the benefits expected out of the procedures and should not guarantee the benefits. For example, subjects participating in exercise training should be informed about the benefit, i.e., achieving better physical endurance status and reducing the risks for diseases but these benefits should not be guaranteed.

Information of Confidentiality

The participants should be informed to maintain confidentiality of the procedures and the information disclosed to them. Authors should give the consent to maintain the confidentiality of the participant's data. The author should state how the data collected from the participant would be processed, where and how it will be published and who all will access it. In case of recording or imaging the subjects, they should be informed about the nature and processing of those data. In the event of disclosure or displaying such recordings and images for publication or presentation, participant permission should be sought prior. The participant should be given the right to review and/or withdraw the consent for permission to display the recordings and images.

Compliance of the Author to Queries

The participant's freedom to ask questions at anytime of the research should be informed. The author should consent to answer the questions raised by the participants at any part of the procedure and answers should be given to the participant's satisfaction.

Consent

Consent of participation should be voluntary. In normal studies, the normal subjects have the right to decide about the participation, in case of patients, they should be informed and assured of the intended treatment if they withdraw from participation. The statement of freedom to withdraw from the study should be included. The participant should be allowed to withdraw from the study at any part of the time, may be in the beginning or during the procedure or even after the data collection (participants withdrawal refers to denial to permit use of their data after collection). The researcher should also state that the procedure may be stopped in due to any unforeseen risks that may occur during the procedure.

Other Elements

Competency of the participant to consent should be assessed. For example, mentally ill patients, children or patients who are critically ill will not be competent to consent. In such situations, consent should be taken from the legal guardian of the participant.

The information and the participants consent to participate in the study should be in writing. The information should be written or comprehended in the participants own language, and consent should be taken after the participant thoroughly understands the information. To overcome legal issues involved it is advised to consider witnesses. The signature part of the written consent should not stand alone on a separate page. Any information which may release the research from legal consideration should be avoided. The mandatory elements of the written informed consent form are stated in the table 7.1.

Table 7.1: Mandatory components of informed consent

1. Statement stating the **rationale and purpose** of the research
2. Detailed explanation of **procedure**
3. Truthful statement of **risks and discomforts** expected in the procedure
4. Description of potential **benefits**
5. **Alternative** procedures might be used
6. Statement to ensure **confidentiality** in process of collection and analyses of patient information, and knowledge of who will access the data
7. Consent to **answer queries and give more information**
8. Statement of participants' right to **refuse or withdraw** without prejudice
9. Description about the management on unforeseen **injuries** and process of dispersion of **compensation**
10. **Consent statement** that participant voluntarily confirms the participation
11. **Signature** of participant/legal guardian and witnesses

The written informed consent form should be taken from all the participants prior to the study. A copy of the written informed consent should be given to the participant. However the participants have a right, not to bind to the consent if he/she believes that the procedure would harm him/her. A sample informed consent form can be found in the annexure for the convenience of the readers.

Institutional Ethical Committee / Institutional Review Board:

The need for the institutional committee to review research was appraised and regulations were made by the World Medical Association at Helsinki in 1975. Helsinki declaration II emphasized that the review of research by Institutional review board should be made mandatory. Institutional ethical committee (IEC) also termed as Institutional review board (IRB) should ensure to safeguard the welfare and rights of human participants in biomedical research. In accordance to international guidelines and Helsinki declaration, the IEC should not only review the research proposal, but also should have regular monitoring for compliance of ethical guidelines by the researcher till the completion of the research.

The IEC should be a multidisciplinary and multisectorial team which ensures the independency and competency of the committee. The IEC should comprise minimum of five members, should not be too large to avoid the difficulty in achieving consensus. The IEC should comprise of Chairman, medical scientist/experts, other professions/clinicians, legal expert, ethicist/theologian, lay person from community and member secretary. The chair person preferably should be from outside the institution to ensure the independency of the committee. The committee should have adequate representation of age, gender, community to safeguard the rights and welfare of all sections of community. All the members should be given freedom to offer views based on societal and cultural norms.

Basic outcomes of the IEC is to protect the rights of research participants; to ensure the compliance of research with ethical guidelines and research standards; and to assist in developing value information of medical research. Responsibilities of IEC are

1. The IEC should review the research proposal and decide on approval or disapproval or modification required during convened meetings
2. Continual review of the project to ensure the welfare and rights of the participants are conserved.

The decision of the IEC should be based on purpose of the study, scientific competency of author(s), risk benefit ratio and feasibility of compliance of the study to ethical guidelines. The IEC should arrive at broad consensus after quorum requirements. The IEC can order to discontinue the project in situations of unequivocal results achieved earlier or non-compliance to ethical guidelines. The IEC may modify, suspend, or terminate approval of research that has been associated with serious harm to subjects or is not being conducted in accord with the IEC's decisions/stipulations/ requirements. The IEC should clearly define the reasons in case of rejection or negative decisions made. By reviewing proposals for research, The IECs also help to protect both the organization and the researcher against potential legal implications of neglecting to address important ethical issues of participants.

Summary

Scientific research done to add information/knowledge to the field of practice, should meet the societal and community needs, and should value the human dignity, rights and welfare. The researcher should have a l responsibility to the community in planning and executing the research, should follow the ethical guidelines put forth by the governing bodies and IEC in their jurisdiction.

Chapter eight

Administration and Management

Leadership is a potent combination of strategy and character. But if you must be without one, be without the strategy

—Gen. H.Norman Schwarzkopf

The ethical issues in management will be considered only at the physiotherapist manager perspective. The broad areas of application of this aspect will be as a health provider- i.e. either in a hospital set up as a middle manager or in a clinic set up, and in academic management. In both of these areas, the manager has a moral responsibility to her employees, to the society and to patients/clients.

IN THE CONTEXT OF HEALTHCARE PROVIDER

Responsibilities to the employee:

In a clinical situation, what responsibility does the employer or the administrating PT have to her staff? The moral values that are an integral part of good management are personal integrity and honesty, fairness and impartiality, a good work ethic, approachability, emotional intelligence, strength of conviction, decision making ability and good interpersonal skills.

Personal honesty and integrity are the cornerstones of good management. A safe, friendly and stimulating working environment is conducive to staff job satisfaction and staff retainment. A good manager is able to balance the needs of her staff with administrative expectations without sacrificing integrity. Specific areas will be dealt with below.

Policy, Procedure, Job Description

The primary duty of a manager towards her staff is to promote communication. To achieve this, clearly defined expectations have to be communicated to the staff at the time of appointment and from time to time thereafter. Flexible duties and policies, aid confusion and chaotic administration. Policy and procedure manuals must be kept at convenient locations and all employees must be required to review them periodically.

Promote Staff-manager Communication

As a manager, the individual has to tread a fine line between policy requirements and the individuality of her staff. Due to the nature of the working conditions of a physiotherapist, which often has to be tailored to suit her patient's needs, there is ample scope for misunderstanding. Let us consider the following example:

The department policy is that all staff must sign in before 9 am. However, the unwritten rule is that 9 am is the outermost limit of sanction and everyone is expected to be at work by 8:30 except in special circumstances. As the head of the department, you notice that a particular staff member, who has been a sincere worker all along, has been signing in consistently at 9 am for the past two weeks. You give her a memo which will go in her employee file. In reply to the memo, she informs you that she has had a patient who due to the medication schedule, has had to be seen from 8 to 9 am which is the reason she has been signing in at 9 am. She was unable to sign in at 8 am as the department opened only at 8:30. This has been unprecedented and you do not have a policy for such a situation.

Both the manager and the staff member are responsible for this debacle. Since it was an unprecedented situation, the staff member should have taken the responsibility of informing the HOD. The HOD in turn should have asked for an explanation before issuing the memo which resulted in unnecessary ill feeling.

As a rule, a manager MUST always seek an explanation prior to issuing any sort of reprimand. This is also the case when giving periodical reports on staff. This is part of the duty of all managers and must be taken seriously. Moreover, a manager must be available and approachable to the staff. Annual reports must have objective, measurable criteria. For example a report that says " xyz is an irresponsible worker" or "xyz is not interested in work" or "xyz is a good worker" without supporting criteria for the statement are all poor and useless reports. To be able to develop a good annual report, the manager must first of all define all policies and procedures of the department, have clear job descriptions for each employee and then formulate a report based on these in a measurable manner, e.g. " xyz is late 50% of the time based on sign –in times for the past year. Hence her punctuality is poor" a reprimand based on this is justified and not challengeable. The temptation for most managers is to toe the middle line and give all staff an average report. This alleviates the need to evaluate carefully and ensures that no employee can accuse the manager of favoritism. However, this is not a desirable course of action as the sincere employees go unnoticed and the poor ones go unreprimanded. This can affect employee morale. Another reason to have an objective policy is to ensure that competence is rewarded. This is also the responsibility of the manager.

All staff who contribute to the department or do their work exceptionally well must be acknowledged. This goes for all staff including janitors, security staff etc. Acknowledgement can be in many ways. The important thing to remember is "always praise in public and reprimand in private".

Safe Working Environment

The provision of a safe working environment is extremely important. This involves the areas of infection control precautions, waste management and equipment safety.

Infection control policies including waste disposal must be clear and strictly followed. This is for the safety of both the employees and the patients. Special care must be taken to educate cleaning staff about potential dangers of coming into contact with infected or dangerous material. Clear areas for disposal of infected material must be designated. Most hospitals have procedures for this and they must be adhered to. Administrators must ensure that masks and gloves are provided for the use of employees and that protective gear is used as per need.

Other aspects of promoting a safe environment, is provision for all prophylactic care, medical care and leave. Probably one of the most important areas for the practicing therapist is education in lifting and transferring. Departments especially rehabilitation units must have provision for mechanical transfer assists to minimize risk of employee injury.

Promote Good Practice

Administrators must encourage their staff to keep up-to-date with advances in their fields by attending continuing education courses etc. Discriminatory practices must be avoided at all costs. All staff must be considered based on their individual merits. Managers must inculcate in their staff a well developed and practical sense of responsibility towards their clients. Transparent policies, will promote a sense of trust and respect towards the manager. This in turn will ensure a lively working atmosphere.

Conflict Management

This is an unpleasant but unavoidable aspect of a manager's job. Individuals will have differences of opinion. It is good management to ensure that these do not flare up into arguments which can cause division and unhealthy competition. Policies must not reward or encourage conflict. This is especially true when unfair advantages are given based on seniority. Although some amount of advantages are earned by seniority, some aspects of policy must be kept uniform. For example all staff irrespective of seniority must be eligible for "employee of the month" awards if there is such a system. All staff must be eligible for continuing education benefits etc. Having clear job responsibilities with clearly demarcated areas is another way to prevent conflict. If conflict does arise, it is necessary to have an unbiased evaluation of the situation. All conflict must be resolved immediately. If not they fester and become unmanageable.

Leave Policy

While it is the privilege of the employee to avail of leave accorded to her, it is the responsibility of the manager to ensure that the departmental needs are not compromised by staff absence. The manager must instill a sense of responsibility in her staff so that they are able to balance the needs of the department with personal needs.

Overtime

It is essential in busy clinics and departments to have a workable overtime policy so that staff do not feel overworked and underpaid. When part of a large organization it is not possible to have separate overtime policies. In this case, the employee's extra work must not go unnoticed. The best solution is to give time off in compensation, which amounts to extra pay.

If even this is not possible, incentives of some sort can be instituted.

RESPONSIBILITIES TO THE PATIENT/CLIENT

Cost Effective Treatment Options

Although this falls under the purview of clinical practice ethics, it is also important in the managerial perspective. Administrative pressure to use certain costlier modalities of treatment in order to recover cost of equipment is not unheard of. While the manager has the responsibility of obtaining only those equipment that are justifiable, it does not condone overuse for economic benefit. The patient has the right to cost effective treatment, which includes time spent. Time spent can be translated to money lost on the part of the patient. This must also be considered. Managerial pressure to continue treating patients when the need is questionable, is highly unethical. As a rule of ethical management, there should be no managerial interference that could cloud a therapist's professional judgement.

Another aspect of responsibility to patients involves equipment. Equipment must be periodically calibrated, serviced and maintained as per manufacturer recommendations. The best way of achieving this is by acquiring "Annual maintenance contracts" for major equipment and ensuring that smaller routine equipment and instruments are regularly serviced by the engineer attached to the clinic. Department policy must stress the habit of routinely testing equipment prior to application on patients.

It is also important to have clear signs and information booklets to avoid undue stress for the patient

Grievance Redressal

Managers must ensure that there is provision of a system where the patient can lodge complaints against the staff members. The best option to improve service is to provide a feedback to assess patient satisfaction. Complaints must be looked into seriously and in an unbiased manner, and action taken upon the merit of these. A similar area is when a patient requests the services of a particular therapist based on previous experience or recommendation from another person, or the gender of the therapist. The best way to handle this is to ensure that the therapists involved have no objection to the change and then acquiesce the patient. If one or both of the therapists object, the issue is best solved by explaining to the patient, that there is a procedure of therapist allocation for administrative ease and then following up to ensure that there are no complaints from the patient about the treating therapist.

OTHER ISSUES

Confidentiality

Confidentiality must be maintained with regard to patient documents as well as employee documents. It shows lack of integrity on the part of the manager to discuss aspects of annual reports with other staff. As much as possible documents of a sensitive nature must be typed by the manager herself to avoid breach of confidentiality that might occur from the secretarial staff. Any patient complaints against a specific therapist or staff must be communicated to the person responsible privately. The same procedure must be followed when one staff member has a complaint against another staff member.

Conflict of Interests

Pharmaceutical companies and equipment companies have been known to offer conditional gifts for purchase of their products. This is a pitfall that must be sidestepped cautiously. Equipment purchases must be conducted based on relative merits and needs of the department.

Use of Photos for Advertisement

If photographs of individuals be it patients or staff are used for advertisements, this must be done only with the prior written consent as it is a breach of confidentiality to do otherwise.

RESPONSIBILITY TO SOCIETY

Any healthcare provider has a moral responsibility to the society at large. It is the duty of a therapist to practice in a way that is beneficial to the society that she serves. Some of the ways that this can be achieved are given below:

Pro bono service: it is good ethical practice to allot a percentage of treatments to be given free of charge or at minimal charge to the economically backward.

Non discriminative practices: while staffing or soliciting clientele, there should be no discrimination. All patients/clients who seek services that are provided by the clinic must be treated equally. This is also important in employment. To avoid any accusations of discriminative practice, it is always best to advertise for positions prominently and then screen candidates in a fair interview.

Objectionable treatment options/clinical trials—this is usually not of application to physiotherapy but rather to drug trials. But there is a chance that drug—electro modality interactions or drug-exercise interactions may occur and companies may be interested in studying these. If there is any participation in such studies by the centre, it is the duty of the manager to adhere to strict protocols of research as outlined in earlier chapters.

Commitment to society—appropriate waste disposal is a major part of the responsibility towards the community. Public awareness programes is another aspect that is the responsibility of healthcare professionals. This is especially true when practicing in areas that are endemic to certain diseases that the PT may have a direct involvement in.

IN THE CONTEXT OF EDUCATIONAL INSTITUTION

Infrastructure, staffing, course structure, examination process, admission process have already been covered substantially in the previous chapter. Certain purely administrative issues will be dealt with here.

PRESSURE TO OBTAIN RESULTS

With academics being a highly competitive business, institutional heads feel pressure to find avenues to project their institutions over others. One of the areas that prospective candidates look at in choice of institution, is their pass percentage in the qualifying examinations. Managers must take care to prevent unscrupulous practices to increase the number of successful students. Unscrupulous practices include coercion of their own staff to give high internal marks in order to offset any low marks being given the external examiner, coercion or bribery of the external examiner to improve the pass percentage, manipulation of results at the university level etc. Needless to say these are all unethical and shows lack of integrity.

Administrative Interference with Examinations

These are instances where the institution promotes cheating at examinations. This may be by means of leaking the paper, handpicking external examiners who are known for their "easy to please" nature, having invigilators who are encouraged to help students cheat etc.

MISCELLANEOUS ISSUES

Traditionally, PT was an offshoot of nursing. In India, this historical fact spawned a number of courses lasting in duration from 3 months to 2 years. This survives in the armed services as well as in civilian hospitals. These courses train the individual to carry out certain routine treatment modalities without reasoning. Hence those individuals who have completed such courses could be considered as an aide or technical assistant to a PT. What would ethical considerations in these cases consist of? Delegation of duties, delegation of patient care responsibilities, and most important how do you deal with a staff of this cadre who has several years of experience? This can be a trying situation for a new graduate who may be intimidated by the sheer fact of age and experience. However, it is the duty of the trained therapist to use the superior theoretical knowledge he/she possesses with the superior experience the aide possesses and strike a happy medium. Easier said than done? Let us consider the following example:

You have recently been appointed as a physiotherapist in a hospital which has previously been staffed by technicians who have been trained on site by the orthopaedics department. These technicians are held in high regard and a certain amount of protectiveness by the orthopaedic department and vice versa. You notice over a period of time that certain treatment modalities may be being overused or other modalities could be used which would be more effective. Other methods are faulty in techniques. You react as follows:

You collect material supporting your observations and approach the orthopaedics consultants and state your cause.

You approach the technician with your evidence and request that maybe the two of you together could make some meaningful changes over time by observing the effects of the correct methods over what has been practiced.

Which is the better option? Obviously the second in many ways! Since the concern is patient care and not discrediting another staff member, taking your justification to anyone else is unnecessary, fosters poor working relations and shows lack of integrity. It is necessary to sort out differences within the department itself.

Next scenario—*you are working in a hospital which has had difficulty retaining the qualified PTs it hires as they all go abroad within a few months to a couple of years. So the administration despite it's best intentions, has now decided that there is no way but to start a short term course, so that these candidates will stay on. They instruct you as the HOD to plan a curriculum of essential knowledge for a PT technician that can be covered in 3 months. You tell them that you will do this only if you are guaranteed that the course will be termed PT aide or technician. They acquiesce. Right ethical conduct?*

Yes if the needs of the hospital and the community it serves justifies this act. Have all other avenues been looked into? Perhaps the reason that the hospital cannot keep its PTs is because of :

1. Low pay
2. Too much interference from administration
3. Too much interference from referring physicians
4. The location of the hospital is too remote.

If the reasons are low pay is it because

A. The hospital is a charitable one and has insufficient financial resources
B. The administration has a condescending opinion of "technical" courses and hence has fixed a low pay scale.

If the reason falls in the first category, you are entirely justified in agreeing to plan and train the short course with the attendant clause that they be given a certificate stating clearly the duration of the course, the designation as aide, the entire syllabus and the objectives of the course which should specify that they are qualified to treat patients only under the supervision of a qualified PT.

If the reason falls into the second category you would be ill advised to comply. However, as you are an employee of the institution, you must try to first of all impress upon the administration your point of view and how it would best serve the patients, the institution, as well as your profession. If this fails, then you have to choose the best course of action. One of these would be to inform the IAP of your dilemma. After that you have to make a moral decision as to whether to comply with the administrative order or quit the job.

If the reason the institution cannot retain it's employees is due to interference from the administration or referring physicians, again your options would be as above. If the reason is due to the remoteness of location, you would be right in planning and executing the course as it would be to the best interest of the community. In this case however you may have to include aspects of care that you may not have in the earlier scenario because you may have to prepare the candidates to work without supervision. So your next dilemma is whether the duration of three months is adequate. Perhaps not. So you would have to convince the administration that the course must be that of a PT assistant and the duration of at least one year.

As you can see, these decisions are not in black and white and finally goes back to the principles of beneficence and distributive justice.

Distance Education

This is a real scenario that requires no hypothetical situations. There are universities conducting distance education courses in every town and village. Is this wholly wrong ? There are parts of the country where there is no accessibility to a good hospital and definitely not to a PT. Considering the special needs of our country- economic as well as access, distance education cannot be totally demonized. Don't people living in remote areas of Arunachal Pradesh have as much right to health care as those people living in Mumbai? Yes. The only practical way may be distance education. Distance education is a means by which large numbers of students can be trained at relatively less cost. The flip side however is this—when the full time student is paying over 10 times the cost and spending a lot more time and finally ends up with the same degree as the distance education candidate, is this situation fair? How do we get around this obstacle? The solution for the previous scenario may hold good here- that the course be that of a PT assistant rather than a PT with compulsory intensive hands on training at designated centers approved of by the IAP. Another option is that the degree certificate specify that the degree was earned through a distance education curriculum.

Continuing Education

Continuing education is a boon as well as a bane to healthcare professions in India. On the one hand, well thought out courses, help to disseminate knowledge and keep professionals up to date on current trends. On the other hand, it may be used as a means of making easy money when in the hands of unscrupulous individuals. Judgement must be used in participating in such courses either as trainers or as delegates.

Summary

Administrators have a responsibility to client, society, employee in the contexts of clinical set up. In the context of education they have a responsibility to the students, society and the employees. Formation of curriculum responsible practice and safety are issues that must be addressed.

Chapter nine

Miscellaneous Issues

The ultimate measure of a man is not where he stands in moments of comfort and convenience, but where he stands at times of challenge and controversy.

- Thomas Jefferson

The previous chapters have dealt with areas of application for ethical practice. In this chapter we shall have a brief look at issues that merit special mention.

Severe Disability

In the Indian scenario with a society where the disabled are fully integrated being a distant dream, and health programs being far from ideal, the role of a physiotherapist falls greatly short of optimum in case of severe chronic disability. A quadriplegic who needs ventilator support for instance has no quality of life in India. He would be confined to a hospital and it would be a great drain on the resources of his family. In this case, the role of the physiotherapist is confined to preventive care, that can easily be carried out by the family or routine nursing care. Hence in such cases, the most empathetic course of action would be to educate the caregivers and withdraw from prolonged routine supportive care.

AIDS

Due to the infections associated with this disease, physiotherapists also become involved in the care of these patients. As the disease is infectious with a high mortality rate, it is essential that infection control precautions are taken stringently. But it is also important to avoid making moral judgements about these patients, and to treat them with compassion. With life expectancy increasing, with appropriate drug therapy it is also important that these patients be considered not as fatal just because of their diagnosis. Appropriate treatment duration must be given.

Hospice Care and Palliative Care

This area is in relation to chronic and fatal disease, notably cancer but also other illnesses like cerebral leukodystrophy etc. While there is very little role in hospice care in India for physiotherapists, this is not the case elsewhere. Pain management and functional independence continue to be a goal even in end of life situations. Is physiotherapy justified in these cases? It is if the patient desires it. If the patient does not, then there is no justification whatsoever.

Chronic Disability

Chronic non fatal disabilities come under the purview of active physiotherapeutic intervention. These situations cause moral dilemmas. The best course of action is to ask oneself the following questions. By continuing therapy, is the patient being given false hope of recovery? Are the visits a drain on the finances of the patient? Is anything being done that is in any way likely to improve the quality of the patients' life? Does the person fully understand the physiotherapy goals?

Based on the answers to these questions the best course of action must be taken. The casuistry approach to ethics is indicated here.

Exposure of Unethical Conduct

What to do when confronted by unethical conduct of one's colleagues or superiors? While it is easy to pontificate on the need to expose unethical conduct, practically the issue is not that clear. There may be extenuating circumstances that you are aware of. The actual incident may be isolated and minor. If you must report whom do you report to? Would it backfire against you? Again there is no stock answer. Ethically speaking, it is at least necessary to make the perpetrator aware of the inappropriateness of her conduct. In the absence of a regulatory body, that is often the best one can do. If the perpetrator is a regular offender, then she must be brought to book either by informing her superiors or the consumer forum if the incidents are harmful to the service recipients. These include immoral acts between therapist and patient.

Placebo Effects

When a certain treatment is known to have only a placebo effect, is application of this treatment to patients ethical? Again this must be considered on a case-by-case basis. Placebo effects which result in improvement in the quality of a patient's life may be justified for short periods of time. Hence the issue of improvement in the quality of life must be ascertained.

Documentation

Treatment note writing is the responsibility of every individual who comes into contact with a patient. These documents must be written clearly with sufficient detail pertaining to services rendered. Unnecessary detail of issues of a personal nature must be avoided. Judgements on the individual must be avoided. Facts must be presented clearly and concisely. The SOAP format is an excellent form of documentation style.

Home Visits

As may be recalled from Chapter II, home visits conducted on the request of an individual fall under the category of a personal contract and as such is not under the purview of the consumer protection act of 1986. Hence these situations put a greater responsibility on the part of the therapist to ensure no misconduct occurs. Home visits must be done only on the request of a patient. Therapists must not solicit these for financial gain. Other options must be offered to the patient and the decision must be made by the patient himself. The other aspect to be considered is the time spent. Care must be taken to spend as much time as one would in a clinic situation. If the treatment offered at home is not optimum or if equipment is required for the patient to obtain maximum benefit, then the patient must be advised to continue treatment at a clinic.

Expert Witness

If called to court to provide a statement when a colleague has been litigated against what is the moral duty of a therapist? Even though the temptation may be to avoid giving contrary opinions, it is necessary to give an honest opinion based on the prevailing knowledge in the area that is of concern. Under the Evidence Act 45, if a person has pursued teaching and training in a specific subject for a specified period following specified norms, he/she can be considered a bona fide witness in the eyes of the law.

Patients of Special Interest

Most therapists have areas that are of special interest to them. In addition, there may be certain patients that are known to them socially or are referred by a physician friend or other similar circumstances. When these patients are routed to another therapist as per policy, what is the best course of action? Obviously it would be most inappropriate to start seeing the patient without the permission or knowledge of the treating therapist. But there is no lack of professional integrity, if the therapist makes it known to her colleagues that certain types of patients should be sent to her because of her special interest in them or that a certain patient is known to her and she would like to see him. However it is the responsibility of the therapist to ensure that no preferential treatment is given just because of her personal interest. If she is unable to have an unbiased relationship with the patient she must hand over to another therapist.

Challenges for the Therapist in India

Regulatory body

The lack of a regulatory body is probably the greatest challenge for a practicing therapist in India. The problems this lapse creates is the absence of norms of behaviour to which one can refer to. Academic guidelines are not uniform throughout the country. Examinations are not uniform, in fact even the course duration is not uniform. Due to this there is a general lack of respect among the physiotherapist fraternity for each other. Standards of care obviously reflect this lack of uniformity. The other aspect is the therapist in India has no one to turn to in case of malpractice suits or even prosecution by her administrators. She is powerless to stop sub standard courses even if she strongly disagrees in principle. The fresh graduate has no resources to seek knowledge. Besides there is an absence of literature being published in India. Western studies do not always have relevance to Indian situations. Problems that are unique to India are seldom addressed. There is no reliable national database that gives information about physiotherapy in India. Many universities that conduct physiotherapy courses do not have any representative from the profession in their board of studies. Other professionals notably physiatrists and orthopaedicians decide what a physiotherapy student must learn. This is obviously far from optimum. Many colleges rely on doctors to take classes in allied subjects. Either the amount of knowledge given is too much and hence the relevance is vague or the teacher keeps emphasising the lack of need for physiotherapy students to learn the topics. This tends to give the student a lack of pride in her profession. If all subjects were taught to undergraduates by academicians who are themselves physiotherapists, perhaps the relevance could be emphasised and the student therapist would have a role model to emulate. Fortunately, the scenario is slowly changing.

Social responsibilities

Another issue unique to India is the prefix "Dr" often used by PTs. Although, IAP mandates that the suffix (PT) must be added, this is often not the case. This may cause confusion in society. Unfortunately there are also miscreants who take advantage of this situation and practice medicine furtively. This issue needs to be considered. Even if the suffix is added, the average citizen assumes that it is a new speciality in medicine. Although the move was made to increase the respectability of the profession, the relevance now is questionable. Perhaps it is time to rethink the issue.

COMMUNITY BASED REHABILITATION

Community based rehabilitation in India is still in its teething stage. The difference from a normal clinical situation is that, here the clients have seldom sought out physiotherapy services. Rather it is the care givers who have sought out clients. In addition to this, CBR requires full and active participation of the community for its wherewithal. The service providers are often performing under stress as they have to show returns to the funding agencies. This being the case, undue coercion or pressure may be laid on the patients/clients. Besides this the other members of the community may also add to the pressure on the disabled. The principle of autonomy must be applied here. Although rehabilitation may be of benefit to the disabled, it is entirely their prerogative whether they want to be rehabilitated or not. Governmental or other goals may have to be met but these targets must not cloud the clinical judgement or moral integrity of the care providers.

Camps

Camps are a common activity of practically every hospital and medical establishment in India. If these are well thought out, adequately staffed and advertised properly, they serve a great purpose. Sadly this is often not the case. Often camps have their sponsors or are done with some ulterior motive mainly promotional.

Hence advertisements often imply benefits or give incomplete information in order to lure more of a crowd. Let us consider the following example:

XYZ physiotherapy college organizes a camp in a rural area which also happens to coincide with the MPT practical examinations. The advertisement states that all people with any ache/ pain/ limp/ any diagnosed or undiagnosed physical problems related to bones, joints, muscles, lungs etc will be evaluated, appropriate measures to alleviate symptoms given and all of these services will be free of cost. The names of certain prominent therapists in the college are printed with the prefix Dr.

There are several problems with this scenario. One of the most obvious is that the college is ensuring that they have adequate patients for MPT examinations. This is unethical as the patients have been lured under false pretences. The second part although true to a physiotherapist, gives a promise of treatment that is more than what will be offered. The names of Drs further strengthens this false impression.

Patients crowd to the camp. At first all patients are received graciously, and screened. Those that are considered appropriate for exams are moved to a separate room and told that a senior Dr will evaluate them shortly. The others are dismissed unceremoniously. The patients used for exams are given an exercise pamphlet and Vit. B complex and analgesic tablets.

Highly unethical again. Since the camp was conducted, it is the moral obligation of the organizers to ensure that all visitors are given due consideration. Those that may be appropriate for MPT examinations must have been asked for their informed consent. Giving of medications even routine, non-prescription drugs is also inappropriate.

A camp that is conducted well, will have some baseline information on the advertising. This should briefly explain what the camp is all about, what physiotherapy can do and make distinctions from doctors so that there is no expectation of medical treatment. It must also explain that only the consultation will be free and any further treatment or referral will be charged. The best way is to not give any promises so that there is no confusion whatsoever. Obviously, there is the possibility of poor attendance. But this risk is better than the alternative strategy.

Patients for Inspection/examination

Many colleges whose affiliated hospitals are small, require patients to fill them during inspection. It is common to fill up beds with chronic patients in return for a payment or other incentive. Likewise for examinations. As practical examinations are conducted on real patients, patients are either called for examinations regularly or ones that are already admitted are kept on. This is inevitable. However, the patient has a right to know the reason for his admission and must not be in any way coerced. If the patient does not want to be part of the examination process, he should be free to go without any implications on his ongoing treatment except that he would forfeit whatever benefits can be given for participating in examinations. It is usually the practice to give a financial incentive by way of reduced hospital charges for those patients who consent for exams. The flip and more humane side of this is the ability to call deserving patients during examinations so that treatment that is required but that they can ill afford can be availed of.

Vulnerable Populations

Special care must be taken when dealing with the old, very young and destitute. This is because these individuals may be unable to give a clear consent or challenge medical decisions. Other parties may make decisions by proxy which may sometimes be in direct conflict with the patient's wishes. It is therefore necessary to ascertain the patient's opinion before a therapist performs treatment. As a rule when the patient is unable to give consent, at least assent for the particular session of treatment must be obtained.

SUMMARY

Issues that need special mention are

Severe disability

AIDS

Hospice care and palliative care

Chronic disability

Exposure of unethical conduct

Placebo effects

Documentation

Home visits

Expert witness

Patients of special interest

Community based rehabilitation

Camps

Use of patients for examinations

BIBLIOGRAPHY AND SUGGESTED READING

1. Business ethics in healthcare- beyond compliance Leonard J Weber, Indiana University Press 2002.
2. Code of Ethical Principles http://nzsp.org.nz/index02/index_Welcome.htm.
3. Ethical guidelines for biomedical research involving human subjects (2000), ICMR Code, ICMR New Delhi.
4. Encyclopaedia Britannica Volume 18 1995.
5. Express healthcare management issue 16-28th February 2003.
6. Gillon R. Ethics needs principles-four can encompass the rest- and respect for autonomy should be "first among equals". Journal of medical ethics July 2005.
7. Guidelines for the conduct of research involving human subjects at national institute of health (2004), US department of Health and human services.
8. http://socialjustice.nic.in/disabled/act.htm.
9. http://www.vakilno1.com/consumer-protect_qns.htm
10. C.M Francis. Medical Ethics, Jaypee 1993.
11. MRC Ethics Guide. Research involving human participants in developing societies, www.mrc.ac.uk
12. Pandya S.K. Issues in medical ethics. Indian Journal of Medical ethics July 2005.

Annexure I

Helsinki II Declaration

INTRODUCTION

It is the mission of the physician to safeguard the health of the people. His or her knowledge and conscience are dedicated to the fulfillment of this mission. The Declaration of Geneva of the World Medical Assembly binds the physician with the words: "The health of my patient will be my first consideration," and the International Code of Medical Ethics declares that, "A physician shall act only in the patient's interest when providing medical care which might have the effect of weakening the physical and mental condition of the patient."

The purpose of biomedical research involving human subjects must be to improve diagnostic, therapeutic and prophylactic procedures and the understanding of the aetiology and pathogenesis of disease. In current medical practice most diagnostic, therapeutic or prophylactic procedures involve hazards. This applies especially to biomedical research.

Medical progress is based on research which ultimately must rest in part on experimentation involving human subjects. In the field of biomedical research, a fundamental distinction must be recognized between medical research, in which the aim is essentially diagnostic or therapeutic for a patient, and medical research, the essential object of which is purely scientific and without implying direct diagnostic or therapeutic value to the person subjected to the research.

Special caution must be exercised in the conduct of research which may affect the environment, and the welfare of animals used for research must be respected. Because it is essential that the results of laboratory experiments be applied to human beings to further scientific knowledge and to help suffering humanity, the World Medical Association has prepared the following recommendations as a guide to every physician in biomedical research involving human subjects. They should be kept under review in the future. It must be stressed that the standards as drafted are only a guide to physicians all over the world. Physicians are not relieved from criminal, civil and ethical responsibilities under the laws of their own countries.

I. Basic Principles

1. Biomedical research involving human subjects must conform to generally accepted scientific principles and should be based on adequately performed laboratory and animal experimentation and on a thorough knowledge of the scientific literature.
2. The design and performance of each experimental procedure involving human subjects should be clearly formulated in an experimental protocol which should be transmitted for consideration, comment and guidance to a specially appointed committee independent of the investigator and the sponsor provided that this independent committee is in conformity with the laws and regulations of the country in which the research experiment is performed.
3. Biomedical research involving human subjects should be conducted only by scientifically qualified persons and under the supervision of a clinically competent medical person. The responsibility for the human subject must always rest with a medically qualified person and never rest on the subject of the research, even though the subject has given his or her consent.
4. Biomedical research involving human subjects cannot legitimately be carried out unless the importance of the objective is in proportion to the inherent risk to the subject.

5. Every biomedical research project involving human subjects should be preceded by careful assessment of predictable risks in comparison with foreseeable benefits to the subject or to others. Concern for the interests of the subject must always prevail over the interests of science and society.
6. The right of the research subject to safeguard his or her integrity must always be respected. Every precaution should be taken to respect the privacy of the subject and to minimize the impact of the study on the subject's physical and mental integrity and on the personality of the subject.
7. Physicians should abstain from engaging in research projects involving human subjects unless they are satisfied that the hazards involved are believed to be predictable. Physicians should cease any investigation if the hazards are found to outweigh the potential benefits.
8. In publication of the results of his or her research, the physician is obliged to preserve the accuracy of the results. Reports of experimentation not in accordance with the principles laid down in this Declaration should not be accepted for publication.
9. In any research on human beings, each potential subject must be adequately informed of the aims, methods, anticipated benefits and potential hazards of the study and the discomfort it may entail. He or she should be informed that he or she is a liberty to abstain from participation in the study and that he or she is free to withdraw his or her consent to participation at any time. The physician should then obtain the subject's freely-given informed consent, preferably in writing.
10. When obtaining informed consent for the research project the physician should be particularly cautious if the subject is in a dependent relationship to him or her or may consent under duress. In that case the informed consent should be obtained by a physician who Is not engaged in the investigation and who is completely independent of this official relationship.

11. In case of legal incompetence, informed consent should be obtained from the legal guardian in accordance with national legislation. Where physical or mental incapacity makes it impossible to obtain informed consent, or when the subject is a minor, permission from the responsible relative replaces that of the subject in accordance with national legislation. Whenever the minor child is in fact able to give a consent, the minor's consent must be obtained in addition to the consent of the minor's legal guardian.
12. The research protocol should always contain a statement of the ethical considerations involved and should indicate that the principles enunciated in the present Declaration are complied with.

II. Medical Research Combined with Clinical Care (Clinical research)

1. In the treatment of the sick person, the physician must be free to use a new diagnostic and therapeutic measure, if in his or her judgement it offers hope of saving life, reestablishing health or alleviating suffering.
2. The potential benefits, hazards and discomfort of a new method should be weighed against the advantages of the best current diagnostic and therapeutic methods.
3. In any medical study, every patient—including those of a control group, if any—should be assured of the best proven diagnostic and therapeutic method.
4. The refusal of the patient to participate in a study must never interfere with the physician-patient relationship.
5. If the physician considers it essential not to obtain informed consent, the specific reasons for this proposal should be stated in the experimental protocol for transmission to the independent committee (I, 2).

6. The physician can combine medical research with professional care, the objective being the acquisition of new medical knowledge, only to the extent that medical research is justified by its potential diagnostic or therapeutic value for the patient.

III. Non-therapeutic biomedical research involving human subjects (Non-clinical biomedical research)

1. In the purely scientific application of medical research carried out on a human being, it is the duty of the physician to remain the protector of the life and health of that person on whom biomedical research is being carried out.
2. The subjects should be volunteers—either healthy persons or patients for whom the experimental designed is not related to the patient's illness.
3. The investigator or the investigating team should discontinue the research if in his/her or their judgement it may, if continued, be harmful to the individual.
4. In research on man, the interest of science and society should never take precedence over considerations related to the wellbeing of the subject.

Annexure II

WCPT Declarations of Principle

DEFINITION

Declarations of Principle record the Confederation's agreed stance on issues affecting the practice of physical therapy internationally and have a two-thirds majority vote thereby becoming policy for all member organisations.

Declarations of Principle

- Ethical Principles.
- Education.
- Protection of Title.
- Primary Health Care.
- Torture.
- Standards of Physical Therapy Practice.
- Quality Care.
- Evidence Based Practice.
- Research.
- Autonomy.
- Private Practice.
- Informed Consent.
- Patients'/Clients' Rights in Physical Therapy.
- Rights of the Client.
- Rights of the Child.
- Relationships with Medical Practitioners.
- Relationships with Other Health Professionals.
- Human Resource Planning.

Physical Therapists

- Respect the rights and dignity of all individuals;
- Comply with the laws and regulations governing the practice of physical therapy in the country in which they work;

- Accept responsibility for the exercise of sound judgement;
- Provide an honest, competent and accountable professional service;
- Are committed to providing quality services according to quality policies and objectives defined by their national physical therapy association;
- Are entitled to a just and fair level of remuneration for their services;
- Provide accurate information to clients, to other agencies and the community about physical therapy and the services physical therapists provide;
- Contribute to the planning and development of services which address the health needs of the community

Declarations of Principle—Education

Physical Therapy education is a continuum of learning beginning with admission to an accredited physical therapy school and ending with retirement from active practice.

- The goal of physical therapy education is the continuing development of physical therapists who are entitled, consistent with their education, to practice the profession without limitation.
- The curricula for physical therapy education should be relevant to the health and social needs of the particular nation.
- The term accredited is used in relation to physical therapy education to describe a program which is regularly evaluated according to established educational standards.
- The first professional qualification should represent completion of a curriculum that qualifies the physical therapist for practice as an independent professional.
- An integral component of the curriculum for the first professional qualification is direct clinical experience under the supervision of appropriately qualified physical therapists. This clinical education will involve gradual access to responsibility
- as skill and experience increase.

- The curriculum should equip physical therapists to practice in a variety of health care settings including, but not limited to, institutional, industrial, occupational and primary health care that encompass urban and rural communities. Consideration should also be given to preparing physical therapists to work in environments that reflect the health care funding models that operate in different countries.
- The curriculum and continuing professional development (CPD) opportunities should prepare physical therapists with knowledge of educational approaches to facilitate the supervision, education and transference of skills to others.
- Life-long learning and professional development is the hallmark of a competent physical therapist. It should be recognised that learning and development may take place in a variety of ways and is not limited to attendance at formal courses.
- Physical therapists should be equipped for evidence-based practice.
- Research methodology should be included in entry-level programs.
- Physical therapists should be encouraged to undertake postgraduate education in physical therapy or related fields for advanced professional development.
- Professional physical therapy education should be conducted by physical therapist-educators able to transfer knowledge and skills about physical therapist examinations/assessment/evaluations, and interventions/treatment and their outcomes, including the critical analysis of theories and methods of physical therapy.
- Basic and foundational sciences (e.g. anatomy, histology, physiology, imaging, etc) and research methodology should be taught by individuals with appropriate education and / or credentials in the area.
- Where national physical therapy associations have adopted practice specialisation, the process to become recognised as a specialist should meet the academic and practice rigors of such a qualification.

- The goals, content, format and evaluation of the education programs provided for physical therapists are the responsibility of the faculty but should involve the active participation of the national physical therapy association.

Declarations of Principle—Protection of Title

The professional names of physical therapy or physiotherapy and the titles physical therapist or physiotherapist, as such or in any translation, are the sole preserve of persons who hold qualifications approved by national professional associations which are members of the World Confederation for Physical Therapy. On behalf of its member organisations, the World Confederation for Physical Therapy claims exclusivity to these titles. Members of the public wishing to access the services of a physical therapist are entitled to know that recognised qualifications are held and that professional behaviour is governed by ethical codes. The World Confederation for Physical Therapy calls on the governments of member organisations to enact legislation, where it does not already exist, to protect the public by limiting the use of these titles to appropriately qualified persons. Further, the World Confederation for Physical Therapy calls on the governments of member organizations to refrain from developing generic classifications that deny the specificity of physical therapy by ensuring that qualified physical therapists always have the right to be employed as physical therapists.

Declarations of Principle—Standards of Physical Therapy

Practice

The World Confederation for Physical Therapy recognises the absolute importance of the development and documentation of agreed standards for the practice of physical therapy. These standards are necessary to:

- demonstrate to the public that physical therapists are concerned with the quality of the services provided and are willing to implement self-regulatory programs to maintain that quality;

- guide the development of professional education; by physical therapists will be consistent with prevailing national quality care standards. Balancing client, organisational and professional considerations, quality care is optimal service at a reasonable cost. Optimal care includes concepts of:
  - equity
  - efficiency
  - effectiveness
  - appropriateness
  - acceptability
  - accessibility ·availability
  - safety.

To obtain this level of optimal care there is a need for:

- Research;
- Development of tools to facilitate evidence-based practice;
- Implementation of evidence and effective change management;
- Evaluation of practice structures, processes and outcomes;
- Monitoring of efficiency, effectiveness and safety;
- Measurement of client satisfaction.

National physical therapy associations must demonstrate leadership in the matter of quality through the development of practice standards and monitoring procedures. They also have a role to play in contributing to the development of multi and uni-professional tools designed to facilitate evidence-based practice, such as clinical guidelines, seeking opportunities for international collaboration where appropriate.

Declarations of Principle—Evidence Based Practice

Physical therapists have a duty and responsibility to use evidence to inform practice and to ensure that the care of clients, their cares and communities is based on the best available evidence. Evidence should be integrated with clinical experience, taking into consideration beliefs and values and the cultural context of the local environment. In addition, physical therapists have a duty and responsibility not to use techniques and technologies that have been shown to be ineffective or unsafe.

Environments that embrace and promote evidence based practice are enabling. Managers and organisations should provide appropriate support structures, resources, facilities and learning opportunities to ensure the delivery of highest quality care. Physical therapists should be prepared to critically evaluate practice. In addition they need to be able to identify questions arising in practice, access and critically appraise the best evidence, and implement and evaluate outcomes of their actions. Relevant life long learning activities are fundamental to evidence based physical therapy and should be introduced in entrylevel physical therapy programs and extended through continuing professional development opportunities. Collaboration both within the profession and with other professions or disciplines is vital to the delivery of evidence based practice. This collaboration needs to take place at a local, national and international level, as appropriate, to facilitate information sharing and best practice, and to capitalise on opportunities for collaborative work that minimises duplication. The WCPT encourages its Member Organizations to develop partnerships and collaborations on projects relevant to evidence based practice. The WCPT and its Member Organisations call on the national governments and non-governmental organisations to facilitate and promote evidence-based healthcare, for example through providing equitable access to the evidence base of health care.

Declarations of Principle—Research

The generation of evidence through research is essential to the development of evidence-based practice in physical therapy. Research in physical therapy should encompass all domains that impact on the practice of physical therapy and client care. This includes, but is not limited to: basic science, diagnosis, specific interventions and technologies [1], service delivery and organisation of care models/systems, economic analysis, development of outcome measures, educational approaches, social-anthropological studies, and health care policy. The most appropriate methods of enquiry should be used to address the topic for research. Research is required that demonstrates clinical and cost effectiveness. It may be necessary to develop and validate new methods of research. Collaboration is critical to the success of any research efforts and the process should include all those who can make a valuable contribution with respect to the initial concept, design, planning, execution, analysis and dissemination. Collaboration is vital within the profession and with other professions or disciplines, as well as with consumers. It needs to take place at the local, national and international level. Physical therapists have a responsibility to promote research efforts and to share freely the results of such research and evaluation through a range of dissemination routes including databases, publication in appropriate professional journals, conference presentations, electronic media and the national press.

Declarations of Principle—Autonomy

The central element of professional autonomy is the assurance that individual physical therapists have the freedom to exercise professional judgement in heath promotion, in prevention and in the care and treatment of clients within the limits of the therapist's prevailing knowledge and competence. In so far as the actions of physical therapists are the responsibility of the individual physical therapists, it follows that their professional decisions cannot be controlled or compromised by employers, persons from other professions or others. As a corollary to the right of professional autonomy, the physical therapy profession has a continuing responsibility to be self-regulating:

- The professional actions and conduct of physical therapists must always be within the bounds of the professional Code of Ethics governing physical therapists in each country;

- National associations must have a procedure for dealing with members who breach the Code, a procedure through which the public may recognise the authority of the profession to regulate itself.

Declarations of Principle—Private Practice

Since physical therapy is an autonomous and independent profession, there should be no impediment to physical therapists entering into a service delivery system, designated private practice, in which individual physical therapists contract to deliver services to the public in accord with government health care policies or market given before any physical therapy is undertaken.

1. A competent adult should be provided with adequate, intelligible information about the proposed therapy:
   - A description of the treatment to be provided;
   - A clear explanation of the risks which may be associated with the therapy;
   - Expected benefits from the therapy; o anticipated time
   - Frames;
   - Anticipated costs;
   - Reasonable alternatives to the recommended therapy.
2. The physical therapist should ensure understanding before seeking consent.
3. When the adult is deemed not competent or when the client is a minor, a legal guardian or advocate may act as a surrogate decision maker.
4. Physical therapists should record in writing in their documentation that informed consent has been obtained.
5. Physical therapists functioning in team situations are responsible for ensuring that appropriate consent arrangements have been made prior to their commencing therapy.

Such collective consent, however, does not negate the physical therapist's responsibility for ensuring that the client is properly informed about the physical therapy.

WCPT Policies—Position Statements

Definition Position Statements reflect the Confederation's preferred opinion on issues affecting the practice of physical therapy and have a simple majority vote. Such statements are available to member organizations to adopt, fully or in part.

Position Statements—Education for Entry-level Physical Therapists

The World Confederation for Physical Therapy recognises the fact that there is considerable diversity in the social, economic and political environments in which physical therapy education is conducted throughout the world. The World Confederation for Physical Therapy recommends that education for entry-level physical therapists be based on university or university level studies, of a minimum of four years, independently validated and accredited as being at a standard that accords graduates full statutory and professional recognition. The World Confederation for Physical Therapy will assist national physical therapy associations with the development of appropriate educational standards and with the development of accreditation processes.

Position Statements—Regulation and Reciprocity

Physical therapy is an internationally recognized health profession which may be practiced by qualified and, where required by state or national legislation, duly registered or licensed physical therapists only. The terms registered / regulation and licensed / licensure are used synonymously. Regulation provides the right to practice physical therapy to the approximately qualified individuals under the appropriate legislative framework. The purpose of regulation is to protect the public from incompetent, unqualified or unethical practitioners. Responsibility for professional regulation varies by country. It may be a government responsibility or a professional responsibility under government legislation or the responsibility of an independent regulatory authority, individual registering authorities develop criteria for entry to physical therapy practice that are specific to the needs of their particular jurisdiction. They also may set continuing competency standards and establish and maintain a process to deal with complaints against members.

Position Statements—Community Based Rehabilitation

Community based rehabilitation (CBR) has been defined as "a strategy within community development for the rehabilitation, equalization of opportunities and social inclusion of all children and adults with disabilities. CBR is implemented through the combined efforts of people with disabilities themselves, their families and communities, and the appropriate heath, education, vocational, and social services."(Draft Joint Position Paper from ILO, UNESCO, UNICEF and WHO, 2002) [1] The World Confederation for Physical Therapy (WCPT) supports the development of CBR as a means of empowering people with disabilities to maximise their physical, mental and social abilities. It recognises that community change is often necessary to promote and fulfil the human rights of people with disabilities to become active participating members of their communities. The WCPT recognises that CBR extends beyond health and encompasses domains such as educational, social, vocational and economic rehabilitation. Inter-agency, cross-sectoral and multi-professional collaboration at all levels is vital in supporting this comprehensive approach to rehabilitation. Health care professionals work with local communities and individuals as partners involved in service planning, operation and monitoring. Physical therapists are equipped to work in both urban and rural settings and have an important contribution to make in CBR:

- By providing interventions aimed at health promotion, disease prevention, treatment and rehabilitation
- By educating and transferring skills to other staff, carers and the community to achieve the fulfillment of physical therapy and client goals

- Through consultancy, advice, support and supervision to other health, education and social care personnel
- As initiators and managers of programs
- As policy advisers to Governments, Non-Governmental Organizations (NGOs) and Disabled People's Organisations (DPOs) Physical therapists are prepared to fulfill these roles through education and continuing professional development opportunities.
- The WCPT calls on national governments and non-governmental organisations to ensure integration in policy development to support CBR. It further calls for equal status to be conferred on those who work in rural communities with those based in urban institutions.

Annexure III

ICMR Code

STATEMENT OF GENERAL PRINCIPLES

Any research using the human beings as subjects of medical or scientific research or experimentation shall bear in mind the following principles:

Principles of essentiality whereby, the research entailing the use of human subjects is considered to be absolutely essential after a due consideration of all alternatives in the light of the existing knowledge in the proposed area of research and after the proposed research has been duly vetted and considered by an appropriate and responsible body of persons who are external to the particular research and who, after careful consideration, come to the conclusion that the said research is necessary for the advancement of knowledge and for the benefit of all members of the human species and for the ecological and environmental well being of the planet.

Principles of voluntariness, informed consent and community agreement whereby, research subjects are fully apprised of the research and the impact and risk of such research on the research subject and others; and whereby the research subjects retain the right to abstain from further participation in the research irrespective of any legal or other obligation that may have been entered into by such human subjects or someone on their behalf, subject to only minimal restitutive obligations of any advance consideration received and outstanding. Where any such research entails treating any community or group of persons as a research subject, these principles of voluntariness and informed consent shall apply, *mutatis mutandis*, to the community as a whole and to each individual member who is the subject of the research or experiment. Where the human subject is incapable of giving consent and it is considered essential that research or experimentation be conducted on such a person incompetent to give consent, the principle of voluntariness and informed consent shall continue to apply and such consent and voluntariness shall be obtained and exercised on behalf of such research subjects by someone who is empowered and under a duty to act on their behalf. The principles of informed consent and voluntariness are cardinal principles to be observed throughout the research and experiment, including its aftermath and applied use so that research subjects are continually kept informed of any and all developments in so far as they affect them and others. However, without in any way undermining the cardinal importance of obtaining informed consent from any human subject involved in any research, the nature and form of the consent and the evidentiary requirements to prove that such consent was taken, shall depend upon the degree and seriousness of the invasiveness into the concerned human subject's person and privacy, health and life generally, and, the overall purpose and the importance of the research.

Principles of non-exploitation whereby as a general rule, research subjects are remunerated for their involvement in the research or experiment; and, irrespective of the social and economic condition or status, or literacy or educational levels attained by the research subjects kept fully apprised of all the dangers arising in and out of the research so that they can appreciate all the physical and psychological risks as well as moral implications of the research whether to themselves or others, including those yet to be born. Such human subjects should be selected so that the burdens and benefits of the research are distributed without arbitrariness, discrimination or caprice. Each research shall include an in-built mechanism for compensation for the human subjects either through insurance cover or any other appropriate means to cover all foreseeable and unforeseeable risks by providing for remedial action and comprehensive aftercare, including treatment during and after the research or experiment, in respect of any effect that the conduct of research or experimentation may have on the human subject and to ensure that immediate recompense and rehabilitative measures are taken in respect of all affected, if and when necessary.

Principles of privacy and confidentiality whereby, the identity and records of the human subjects of the research or experiment are as far as possible kept confidential; and that no details about identity of said human subjects, which would result in the disclosure of their identity, are disclosed without valid scientific and legal reasons which may be essential for the purposes of therapeutics or other interventions, without the specific consent in writing of the human subject concerned, or someone authorised on their behalf; and after ensuring that the said human subject does not suffer from any form of hardship, discrimination or stigmatisation as a consequence of having participated in the research or experiment.

Principles of precaution and risk minimisation whereby due care and caution is taken at all stages of the research and experiment (from its inception as a research idea, its subsequent research design, the conduct of the research or experiment and its applicative use) to ensure that the research subject and those affected by it are put to the minimum risk, suffer from no irreversible adverse effects and, generally, benefit from and by the research or experiment; and that requisite steps are taken to ensure that both professional and ethical reviews of the research are undertaken at appropriate stages so that further and specific guidelines are laid down, and necessary directions given, in respect of the conduct of the research or experiment.

Principles of professional competence whereby, the research is conducted at all times by competent and qualified persons who act with total integrity and impartiality and who have been made aware of, and are mindful of, the ethical considerations to be borne in mind in respect of such research or experiment.

Principles of accountability and transparency whereby, the research or experiment will be conducted in a fair, honest, impartial and transparent manner after full disclosure is made by those associated with the research or experiment of each aspect of their interest in the research, and any conflict of interest that may exist; and whereby, subject to the principles of privacy and confidentiality and the rights of the researcher, full and complete records of the research inclusive of data and notes are retained for such reasonable period as may be prescribed or considered necessary for the purposes of post-research monitoring, evaluation of the research, conducting further research (whether by the initial researcher or otherwise) and in order to make such records available for scrutiny by the appropriate legal and administrative authority, if necessary.

Principles of the maximisation of the public interest and of distributive justice whereby, the research or experiment and its subsequent applicative use are conducted and used to benefit all human kind and not just those who are socially better off but also the least advantaged; and in particular, the research subject themselves.

Principles of institutional arrangements whereby, there shall be a duty on all persons connected with the research to ensure that all the procedures required to be complied with and all institutional arrangements required to be made in respect of the research and its subsequent use or application are duly made in a bonafide and transparent manner; and to take all appropriate steps to ensure that research reports, materials and data connected with the research are duly preserved and archived.

Principles of public domain whereby, the research and any further research, experimentation or evaluation in response to, and emanating from such research is brought into the public domain so that its results are generally made known through scientific and other publications subject to such rights as are available to the researcher and those associated with the research under the law in force at that time.

Principles of totality of responsibility whereby the professional and moral responsibility, for the due observance of all the principles, guidelines or prescriptions laid down generally or in respect of the research or experiment in question, devolves on all those directly or indirectly connected with the research or experiment including the researchers, those responsible for funding or contributing to the funding of the research, the institution or institutions where the research is conducted and the various persons, groups or undertakings who sponsor, use or derive benefit from the research, market the product (if any) or prescribe its use so that, inter alia , the effect of the research or experiment is duly monitored and constantly subject to review and remedial action at all stages of the research and experiment and its future use.

Principles of compliance whereby, there is a general and positive duty on all persons, conducting, associated or connected with any research entailing the use of a human subject to ensure that both the letter and the spirit of these guidelines, as well as any other norms, directions and guidelines which have been specifically laid down or prescribed and which are applicable for that area of research or experimentation, are scrupulously observed and duly complied with. These 12 principles laid down under Statement on General Principles are common to all areas of biomedical research. The specific issues are mentioned under relevant topics.

Annexure IV

Sample Consents

A) SAMPLE INFORMED CONSENTS

COLLEGE OF PHYSIOTHERAPY, XYZ UNIVERSITY, SRIRANGAPURAM

Title of research study: Treatment of PA shoulder
Principal investigator: Leelavathi P.

Participants Name: **Hosp. No.:**

Purpose of research:

I have been informed that this study will test the effectiveness of two different physiotherapy treatments for treating shoulder pain and stiffness. Both are accepted forms of therapy. This study will help physiotherapists understand which of the two methods is more useful in patients who have similar problems.

Procedure

I understand that I will be assigned by lot to either of two groups- one consisting of appropriate modalities for pain relief and conservative exercise protocol ad the other of appropriate modalities for pain relief and manual therapy procedures. Neither procedure requires me to be hospitalized nor are the charges for them different. In addition to the exercises, I will be subjected to evaluation procedures by the physiotherapist.

Risks and Discomforts

I understand that I may experience some pain or discomfort during the course of examination and treatment. These are due to the nature of my condition and the physiotherapy procedures are not expected to exaggerate the symptoms associated with my condition.

Benefits

I understand that as a result of my participation in this study I will have no benefit given to me other than the potential relief of my symptoms. The major benefit expected is to find out which treatment program is superior.

Alternatives

I understand that the two physiotherapy programs offered as part of this study are standard physiotherapeutic measures for my condition. There are no other physiotherapy alternatives offered by this department.

Confidentiality

I understand that medical information produced as a result of this study will become part of my permanent medical records and will be subject to the confidentiality and privacy regulations of the hospital. Information of a sensitive nature will not be included in the records.

If the data is used for publication, or for teaching purposes, no names or other identification will be given.

Request for More Information

I understand that I may at any time request more information about the study and about my condition and progress. I will be informed about any significant new information that may affect me or influence my further participation in the study.

Withdrawal from the Study

I understand that I may at any time withdraw from the study without explanation. My participation is completely voluntary and will have no bearing on my continued treatment in the department. I also understand that the investigator may terminate my participation in this study at any time after she has explained the reasons to my satisfaction, and has arranged for my continued care.

Injury Statement

I understand that in the unlikely event of any untoward incident occurring as a direct result of my participation in this study, I will be accorded of medical treatment to alleviate the symptoms. I understand that by my agreement to participate in this study, I am not waiving any legal rights.

Investigator's Statement

I have explained to ——————————, the purpose of the research, the procedures required, and the possible risks and benefits to the best of my ability.

Investigator   Date

I confirm that —— has explained to me all the details of the proposed study. I consent to participate with full understanding of the procedures.

Participant   Date

Witness   Date

B) SAMPLE INFORMED CONSENT (Alternative)

COLLEGE OF PHYSIOTHERAPY, XYZ UNIVERSITY, SRIRANGAPURAM

Title of research study: Treatment of PA shoulder
Principal investigator: Leelavathi P.

Participants Name: **Hosp. No.:**

Purpose of Research

Purpose of this study is to test the effectiveness of two different physiotherapy treatments for treating shoulder pain and stiffness. Both are accepted forms of therapy. This study will help physiotherapists understand which of the two methods is more useful in patients who have similar problems.

Procedure

You will be assigned by lot to either of two groups- one consisting of appropriate modalities for pain relief and conservative exercise protocol and the other of appropriate modalities for pain relief and manual therapy procedures. Neither procedure requires you to be hospitalized nor are the charges for them different. In addition to the exercises, you will be subjected to evaluation procedures by the physiotherapist.

Risks and Discomforts

You may experience some pain or discomfort during the course of examination and treatment. These are due to the nature of your condition and the physiotherapy procedures are not expected to exaggerate the symptoms associated with your condition.

Benefits

As a result of your participation in this study you will have no benefit given other than the potential relief of your symptoms. The major benefit expected is to find out which treatment program is superior.

Alternatives

The two physiotherapy programs offered as part of this study are standard physiotherapeutic measures for your condition. There are no other physiotherapy alternatives offered by this department.

Confidentiality

The medical information produced as a result of this study will become part of your permanent medical records and will be subject to the confidentiality and privacy regulations of the hospital. Information of a sensitive nature will not be included in the records. If the data is used for publication, or for teaching purposes, no names or other identification will be given.

Request for More Information

You may at any time request more information about the study and about your condition and progress. You will be informed about any significant new information that may affect you or influence your further participation in the study.

Withdrawal from the Study

You may at any time withdraw from the study without explanation. Your participation is completely voluntary and will have no bearing on your continued treatment in the department. I may terminate your participation in this study at any time after explaining the reasons to you, and arrangements will be made for your continued care.

Injury Statement

In the unlikely event of any untoward incident occurring as a direct result of your participation in this study, you will be accorded medical treatment to alleviate the symptoms. By your agreement to participate in this study, you have not waived your legal rights.

Investigator Date

I confirm that (Investigator) has explained to me all the details of the proposed study. I consent to participate with full understanding of the procedures.

Participant Date

Witness Date

